Springer Series on Medical Education

Carole J. Bland, PhD, Series Editor
Steven Jonas, MD, Founding Editor

Peggy Wallace, PhD, is Associate Adjunct Professor of Medicine and Director of Curricular Resources and Clinical Evaluation at the University of California, San Diego School of Medicine, where she is responsible for the teaching, assessment, and remediation of clinical skills using standardized patients in the undergraduate medical school curriculum. For the past 10 years she has been Director of the Professional Development Center at the UCSD School of Medicine, where the clinical skills of residents and practicing physicians are also being assessed. Before entering the field of medical education, she studied music and dance, did graduate work in instructional media, cinema, and television, and then was hired at the University of Southern California (USC) to operate the first computer-based manikin used to train anesthesiology residents. This beginning in medical simulation ultimately led to her work with standardized patients.

Dr. Wallace held a faculty position at USC in the Department of Medical Education under Dr. Stephen Abrahamson from 1977 to 1995 and was responsible, along with Dr. Howard Barrows, for the reintroduction of standardized patients into the USC Medical School curriculum beginning in the mid-1980s. In the early 1990s, Dr. Wallace became one of the founding directors of what ultimately became the California Consortium for the Assessment of Clinical Competence (CCACC), a consortium of all eight medical schools in California. She is currently codirector of the CCACC whose purpose is the design and yearly administration of a high-stakes Clinical Practice Examination given to all senior medical students in the state of California. She has initiated and participated in research within the CCACC to determine and improve standardized patient performance in case presentation and checklist accuracy, as well as designed an effective remediation program for students who do not perform up to the expected standards on the communication skills component of clinical performance examinations at UCSD. She has served as consultant to the National Board of Medical Examiners on the Standardized Patient Project, which produced the USMLE Step 2 Clinical Skills Examination. Additionally, Dr. Wallace has conducted numerous workshops nationally, and for the World Health Organization internationally, on instructional technology, the use of video in medicine, procedures for training standardized patients, and SP case development. She has also published a history of the use of standardized patients in medical education entitled *Following the Threads of an Innovation.*

Coaching
Standardized Patients

For Use in the Assessment of
Clinical Competence

Peggy Wallace, PhD

Best wishes
Peggy Wallace
7/08

SPRINGER PUBLISHING COMPANY
NEW YORK

Springer Publishing Company, LLC
11 West 42nd Street, 15th Floor
New York, NY 10036

Acquisitions Editor: Sheri W. Sussman
Managing Editor: Mary Ann McLaughlin
Production Editor: Matthew Byrd
Cover Design: Joanne E. Honigman
Composition: Techbooks

07   08   09   10/5   4   3   2   1

Library of Congress Cataloging-in-Publication Data

Wallace, Peggy.
    Coaching standardized patients : for use in the assessment of clinical
competence / Peggy Wallace.
        p. ; cm. – (Springer series on medical education)
    Includes bibliographical references and index.
    ISBN 0-8261-0224-7 (hardback)
    1. Nursing–Study and teaching.   2. Clinical competence–Evaluation. I.
Title. II. Series: Springer series on medical education (Unnumbered)
    [DNLM: 1. Education, Medical–methods.   2. Patient Simulation.
3. Clinical Competence.   4. Teaching–methods. W 18 W193c 2007]
RT71.W35 2007
610.73076–dc22

                                                                    2006017057

Printed in the United States of America by Bang Printing.

To

Stephen Abrahamson,   *and*   Howard S. Barrows,
"the king" who hired me   without whom none of us
into his realm   would be doing this work
Grâce à Sim I . . .   *Namaste . . .*

all the standardized patients and SP educators with whom
I have had the privilege of working throughout the years

and

all who continue to bring their talent and insight
into a process that is shaping the learning of clinical skills
in medical schools across North America and around the world.

Contents

Contents

List of Figures and Tables

Preface

Many times over the years I have found myself musing about how I ended up working in medicine. On the one hand, my father was a physician, but he discouraged me from following in his footsteps. It was the era when we were told "that's not a good profession for a woman"—like so many other professions that were not for women in the early 1960s. On the other hand, because I was a young woman, I was free to pursue pretty much anything else I was interested in, which left me free to go where I was being led—to music, to dance, and eventually to film. As I look back on it all, I see the theme I couldn't see at the time—the longing to express the inexpressible and the need to heal the emotional wounds that are part of being human. So I sought the safety of the halls of academe, pursuing degrees in those three areas, one after another, discovering along the way that I like to teach—and pursuing that as well. By the time I had finished the degrees, I couldn't find a suitable job. . . until one day (I'm still amazed), something urged me to walk into the Department of Medical Education at the University of Southern California in 1979 and ask if they might have a job for me. And they did. Someone had just precipitously quit, so I was hired to run Sim I, the first computer-operated manikin that was then being used to train anesthesiologists. I was only hired for 6 months, but 5 years later I was still there when Dr. Howard Barrows was invited back to USC (the very place he first started to use standardized patients) to reestablish their use in the medical school curriculum. I was put in charge of this effort because I had a background in instructional media, and they thought I knew something about working with actors—which I did not. So I ended up working in medicine after all, supporting students as they learn to listen to their patients' deepest concerns and helping faculty physicians train each new class of aspiring doctors.

Now, why have I told you this story? Simply to say that if you find yourself working with standardized patients, something has led you

there—some desire, some quirk of fate, some longing perhaps to participate in some kind of healing yourself.

THE EVOLUTION OF THIS BOOK

For a number of years, with the encouragement of some of my colleagues, I
considered putting in writing what it is that we do as standardized patient
coaches, based on my own experience. The methods and procedures in this
book have evolved over the past 25 years and have essentially come from
working with Howard Barrows, MD, and Stephen Abrahamson, PhD
(one of the fathers of medical education), who together initiated the work
to establish standardized patient-based clinical performance examinations
in U.S. medical schools in order to effect broad-based curricular change.
These methods and procedures have also grown out of working with
the members of the National Board of Medical Examiners' Standardized
Patient Subcommittee, who represented the University of Massachusetts,
the University of Connecticut, Southern Illinois University, the University
of Texas Medical Branch at Galveston, and the University of Manitoba—
and, of course, my longstanding work with the SP coaches from the eight
medical schools that compose the California Consortium for the Assessment of Clinical Competence (CCACC).

THE PURPOSE OF THIS BOOK

Because the purpose of this book is to describe and codify some of the best
practices and most skillful methods coaches use when preparing standardized patients (SPs)[1] to perform in high-stakes clinical skills examinations,
the coaching methods you will find in this book are designed to produce
the highest standards of SP performance authenticity and the highest accuracy in the SPs' patient portrayals and in their checklist recording. You
will also find information to help you coach your SPs into writing the
most effective feedback so that the scores that the medical students get on
their communication skills have more specific relevance to them—rather
than numbers alone—in terms of what the "patient" experienced in the
clinical encounter with them.

---

[1] A standardized patient is a person who is carefully trained to accurately, repeatedly, and realistically re-create the history, physical findings, and psychological and emotional responses
of the actual patient on whom the case is based so that anyone encountering that "patient"
experiences the same challenge from the SP, no matter when the case is performed or which
of the SPs trained to portray the case is encountered.

After writing this book, I am more aware than ever before of just how remarkable, unique, and intricate are the combined skills required to do this work of coaching standardized patients. For the past decade, events in the United States, Canada, several European countries, and elsewhere in the world have been prodding SP coaches to organize ourselves (witness the growth of our own international professional organization, the Association of Standardized Patient Educators [ASPE]), to systematize and define the basic, necessary elements of the SP training discipline, and to research which methods work best and under which circumstances.

As a reader, you might be an experienced SP coach, or you might be new to this discipline. You might be working with medical students or students of pharmacy, nursing, chiropractic, physician's assistant, social work, counseling psychology, family therapy, or law, to name a few of the fields in which this kind of human simulation methodology is used for teaching, assessment, and certification purposes. You might be a clinical researcher or a faculty member who wants to understand what is involved in the preparation of SPs for their work in the assessment of clinical competence. No matter what your situation is, it is my hope that you will find ideas, techniques, or principles that will expand and deepen your understanding of both the art and the practice of coaching SPs. Whatever your purpose in reading this book, it is my intent that you come to understand more deeply the importance of the skills of the coach and the precision of the work necessary for your trainees to consistently produce performances that are authentic, checklists that are accurate, and feedback that is effective.

THE BROADER APPLICATIONS OF THIS BOOK

Although the contents of this book pertain to the most rigorous type of recruitment, auditioning, selection, and training procedures necessary to assure the highest quality patient simulations for the assessment of clinical competence, there are less demanding circumstances in which the use of standardized patients is both desirable and appropriate, such as in teaching and learning scenarios. If it is understood that the principles, the process, and the guidelines for the recruitment, auditioning, selection, and training of standardized patients remain fundamentally the same, then one can safely adapt the details of the procedures found in this book to fit the various learning activities in which an SP might be needed as an essential component.

Are the skills and methods described in this book the only way to ensure high-quality SP performances? Certainly not. The methods I have shared here are not intended to be the final word on SP coaching. There is no *one* right way. My hope is, however, that this book will be of service to you, especially if you are an SP coach, and that it may be a vehicle by which you discover your way, your path—the one that supports you in finding the skillful means that work specifically for you and your SPs.

Acknowledgments

I want to thank

Karen Garman without whose ever-present personal support and professional coaching this book would not be in your hands.

Anita Richards and Robert MacAulay from whose remarkable talents I have learned much and whose faith in what I was doing often gave me the courage I needed to continue.

Diane Richards and Vivian Hercules who held down the fort with style and aplomb in my absence.

Bryan Bevell who coached me, beyond generosity, to understand what on earth it was I was doing intuitively that he could do with such keen awareness.

Judy Barclift, Sarah Dempster Hall, Romy Kitrell, Robert MacAulay, and Anita Richards, all of whom read parts or all of the manuscript and helped me see what was needed with fresh eyes.

Melinda Schwakhofer and Angela Atencio, the SP educators who companioned me in the early days when none of us really knew what we were doing.

All of the members of the Standardized Patient Sub-Committee at the National Board of Medical Examiners, an amazing group of professionals with whom I had the privilege of working. Thanks to Ann King, Michelle Marcy, Mary Philbin, Linda Perkowski, Carol Pfeiffer, and Gail Schnabel.

The original SP educators of the California Consortium for the Assessment of Clinical Competence—Sue Ahearn, Becky Bartos, Camille Fitzpatrick, Nancy Heine, Ellen Lewis, and Elizabeth O'Gara—who participated in the initial refinement of the training procedures we are using in the CCACC. I am grateful to them and to all the SP educators in the CCACC for their dedication to the quality of our coaching and for their ongoing creative ideas that are contributing to the advancement of SP coaching methodology.

Michael Prislin, friend and colleague, who, by his example in our professional work together, demonstrated the value of transparency in leadership.

Emil Petrusa for sharing with me his considerable insight into the research that has been done on clinical performance assessment.

Andres Sciolla and Linda Perkowski for their words of encouragement that always seemed to come just when they were most needed.

Gloria Avrech who helped me to recognize over and over throughout the years that the feminine has its own rhythm, its own way of unfolding.

Kent Smith who, in a golden circle of fallen gingko leaves under a full moon, wrote to wish me ease with the writing.

Phyllis Barrows who constantly emailed me, giving me the courage I needed in the beginning to believe I could write this book.

Jon Snyder who brought me "meals on wheels"—up to the very end.

Felix Sui who remained a faithful friend, encouraged me to see that time away from writing was a good thing, not a reason for guilt—and fixed my computer to boot.

Walt Young who taught me to play the didjeridoo and helped me see that playing and dancing could free up the writing.

Carol Pfeiffer who reminded me that a well-crafted rowboat might be all that's needed—even when there's a temptation to build an ocean liner.

Sheri W. Sussman whose patience and faith in my finishing the book brought it into print just in the nick of time.

Hazel Hunley, humorist *par excellence*, whose wisdom and editorial insights are reflected in every nook and cranny of this book.

Wicca, my ever-constant companion, who kept me company through the many hours of isolation it took to put my thoughts and experiences on paper.

And to the spirit of White Crow Woman....

Introduction

THE MAKING OF A DISCIPLINE

Two nearly simultaneous occurrences in the early 1990s in the United States have helped shape our SP training into a professional discipline. First, the National Board of Medical Examiners worked diligently to put the SP-based clinical skills performance assessment into the United States Medical Licensure Examination, and second, the Josiah Macy, Jr., Foundation funded and thereby challenged a number of strategically placed medical school consortia throughout the United States to design clinical skills examinations using standardized patients. The premise of the Macy Foundation support was that if the means to actually measure the medical students' level of clinical competence was placed in the curriculum in a number of medical schools, and if faculty could statistically see how students were actually performing on the clinical skills they were acquiring, it would drive the curricular changes that seemed necessary in medical education at the end of the 20th century.

As our discipline has evolved, the coaching that we do with standardized patients has evolved as well and now requires us to blend many skills. We must have the ability to find, audition, and select the right people to play the patients. We must make sure that our SPs learn the facts and deliver them at the appropriate time in the clinical encounters, as well as assure that they can accurately perform the simulated physical findings of the patient they are portraying. We must guide them in understanding each item of the case checklist and make sure that they can observe and recall what happened in the encounter so that their completion of each checklist item is accurate. We must coach them how to write effective feedback on the examinee's interaction skills. We must do all this while supporting the SPs' efforts to make the patient's reality their own in such a way that their performances subtly, but palpably, communicate the complexity of what it means for a patient to be vulnerable and human. This book focuses on all of these coaching skills in the context of training the SPs to work in high-stakes clinical skills examinations, which requires of the SPs the most authentic and precise performance standards.

THE EXACTING DEMANDS OF SP WORK

In order to accurately assess a medical student's clinical skills, that is, his or her ability to take a medical history, perform an appropriate physical examination, and educate or inform patients about their condition in a respectful, caring, and relationship-centered manner, the student must be observed working with patients. Clinical skills cannot be assessed with a written test of the student's cognitive knowledge. In other words, tests of knowledge cannot assess how effectively the students can incorporate their medical knowledge into clinical practice. In fact, any skill that cannot be judged by a written exam, such as playing a musical instrument or competing in gymnastics, must be evaluated by observation of the performance itself. This is true of the medical students' clinical skills as well.

Performance assessment is usually done by an expert or a jury of experts who observe and evaluate a performer's skills. In medicine, the students are supposed to be assessed during their years of intensive clinical skills training through observation by various faculty physicians, the experts whose role it is to evaluate the student's acquisition of clinical skills as they progress from one clerkship to another. However, because of the increasing responsibilities in their clinical research and medical practices, it is difficult for faculty physicians to find time to directly observe and assess the medical students' clinical skills because both the faculty and students are often working simultaneously with separate patients. It was partly out of the need for this direct observation of students in medical training that the clinical skills performance examination using standardized patients was born in the 1980s—and it is one of the reasons that these SP-based examinations have had such staying power. In essence, the SPs have become surrogate observers who are responsible for accurately recording the medical students' clinical behaviors so that the faculty physicians can determine by the students' exam scores if they are performing up to the standards expected of them. Consequently, it has become the SP coach's remarkable responsibility to train the standardized patients to stand in for the faculty physicians as observers of the medical students' clinical skills performances.

Because the direct observation and assessment of the medical student's interactions with patients is increasingly done by standardized patients, let's consider the uniqueness of what is required of them.

Standardized patients, who more often than not have no background in medicine, must not only simultaneously perform the role of the patient while interacting with the medical student, but must also observe and then recall accurately what the student did during the clinical encounter. In addition, while completing the case checklist,[1] the SP must interpret each item as it has been defined by the physician experts who designed the checklist, but who are not usually present during the clinical examinations. This is a role of great consequence that the SPs are taking on and a huge responsibility for the coaches training them because of the necessity for obtaining accuracy in the data that the SPs submit on the student's clinical performances. Given all of this, the question arises: Is it possible for SPs to be 100% accurate on the checklist? Yes, it is. Can we be certain that the SPs' data on the medical students' performances will be 100% accurate all of the time—as are the data on a student's written test of knowledge? No, we cannot. But, amazing as it seems, we *are* certain from the research that has been done that SPs can be consistently accurate at a high enough level for these clinical skills performance tests to determine which examinees meet the minimum level of competence established by the medical faculty (Colliver & Williams, 1993). However, there is a caveat with this statement: SPs can be consistently accurate enough *only if* they are selected well, trained to the highest standards, and then monitored and given feedback on their portrayals and their checklists throughout their training and during all of the administrations of the clinical skills examination. Otherwise, no one can be certain how accurate the numbers are in the data that were collected.

Therefore, the most exacting kinds of recruitment and training of standardized patients are required for high-stakes clinical skills examinations, whether they be used to assess the progress of health care professionals in training or to recertify practicing clinicians throughout their careers. This kind of summative performance examination is known by several names. The National Board of Medical Examiners calls their high-stakes licensure exam the Step 2 CS (Clinical Skills) Examination, whereas in medical schools it is variously known as the Clinical Skills Assessment (CSA), Clinical Competence Exam (CCE), Clinical Performance Exam, or generically as Objective Structured Clinical Examinations (OSCEs), to name a few. In this book, I use the term Clinical Practice Examination (CPX) to refer to these high-stakes assessments because in such examinations students are expected to see a number of standardized patients,

---

[1] Each patient case portrayed by the SPs has its own checklist of items that the SPs fill out, documenting what the medical student (the examinee during an actual exam) has done in the course of the interaction with them as the patient.

one after another in a clinical setting, just as primary care physicians see patients in their clinical practices. These types of examinations are usually given to students shortly after they have completed all of their required clinical clerkships.

The high-stakes nature of this type of exam has to do with the consequences attached to it. For instance, many medical schools make it a requirement that students achieve a passing grade on such performance-based examinations as a condition for graduation. Although standardized clinical performance examinations are not without flaws, no other method currently available has been proven to be as effective as these SP-based examinations for assessing the clinical skills of health care professionals in training (Colliver & Williams, 1993; Petrusa, 2002). This places an enormous responsibility on the faculty who design the overall structure of the performance-based examinations and develop the patient cases, on those who coach the SPs, and on the SPs themselves—a responsibility that has long-range implications for graduating well-qualified medical professionals.

DEFINING COACHING

For years, those of us who have been working with SPs have been called trainers. Even the Association of Standardized Patient Educators defines its mission as providing "support, resources and educational opportunities to medical educators involved in SP methodology, from deans and medical directors to teaching and support faculty, program coordinators, and standardized patient trainers." (See www.aspeducators.org). I have no objection to the term *trainer*. In fact, the synonyms for trainer (educator, instructor, preceptor, tutor, and coach) overwhelmingly affirm our role as a teacher.

Certainly these synonyms apply to SP work, but to me the nuances of the word *coach* capture better than any other the essence of how I envision our work. For instance, a coach often has a special relationship with his or her protégé, no matter what field: sports, opera, dance, business, SP work. The coach puts the performance of her protégé above her own self-interest. Coaches get their satisfaction out of how well their charges are doing. Coaches symbolically, and often literally, stand alongside their protégés and cheer them on. Coaches are aware of the differences among their charges and find their challenges in figuring out how best to maximize the strengths of each. In fact, coaches will do anything necessary—teach, nudge, support, encourage, run interference—to make sure their charges succeed. From both sides of the equation, what is important is the relationship between the coach and the protégé and the fact that the emphasis is on the protégé's success in achieving the goal he is working toward. All of these descriptions of a coach taken collectively are how I see us working with our SPs. I know that those of you already working with standardized patients know the special relationship I am talking about. But whatever we decide to call ourselves, what matters most is *how* we do what we do, the spirit in which we do it, and the outcomes we see in our SPs' performances, which result from the multiple ways we have been able to motivate and bring out the best in each of them.

AN OVERVIEW OF THE BOOK

This book can be read from cover to cover, of course, but it can also be used as a reference so that you can go to particular sections when you need them while you are training your SPs.

The book is laid out in two parts. Part One encompasses the skills and knowledge necessary to do a thorough job of coaching. It contains an in-depth description of specific ways to develop or add to your repertoire of skills if you are already an SP coach, or to start developing these skills if you are a beginning SP coach. Part Two provides information on how to find the right SP along with specific procedures you can use to train your standardized patients. It outlines the SP training program in which you can incorporate many of the skills and techniques discussed in Part One.

The four chapters in Part One focus on the specific skill sets and knowledge that an SP coach must have or acquire in order to assist the SPs in producing realistic performances of the patients they are portraying. Chapter 1 provides an overview of standardized patient coaching. Chapter 2 acquaints coaches who do not have a background in medicine with a number of ways to acquire the essential clinical or "doctoring" skills needed to perform the role of the medical student when training their SPs to portray the patient. Chapters 3 and 4 provide the coach with some background in the dramatic arts, information that is important when coaching the SPs to realistically portray the patient's emotional and psychological qualities. Chapter 3 focuses on the fundamentals and techniques of acting that a coach needs to understand in order to help the SPs create true-to-life performances of the patient case. Chapter 4 is about directing, including techniques for coaching the SPs to give performances that match the coach's vision of the patient being portrayed.

Part Two offers specific methods and procedures to find the right SPs to play the patients during the CPX and to train them to perform at the highest level possible to assure that the data the SPs report (which determine the students' exam scores) are highly accurate in representing the medical students' actual clinical performances. Each chapter in Part Two describes the practical and sequential steps of SP training including the training procedures themselves. Chapter 5 covers the steps for recruiting the best SPs to play the patient case—a critical task, because if poor choices are made in the selection of the SPs, the coach is in for trouble from the start. Chapter 6 contains an overview of what is involved in training the recruits to get ready to perform as standardized patients in CPX-type examinations. Chapters 7 through 10 contain a specific set of detailed procedures for coaches to use in sequence when training their SPs. Chapter 11 describes variations on the four training session protocols, suggesting other possibilities for mixing and matching different aspects of training in order to assist the SPs in acquiring the different skill sets. Finally, Chapter 12 presents the procedures for the Practice Exam, which in essence is a mock-up of an actual CPX administration. During the Practice Exam the SP coaches have a chance to monitor their SPs and give them last-minute feedback on their performances before they start working with the medical students in the actual exam.

OTHER RESOURCES IN THE BOOK

Appendix A contains a full set of documents for the Maria Gomez standardized patient case, which is referred to as a representative example throughout the book. This case has been piloted, revised, and used in multiple clinical skills assessments of third-year medical students at the University of California, San Diego.

The case of Maria Gomez[2] is based on a real patient in the clinical practice of the case author, Dr. Stacie San Miguel, a family medicine physician on the UCSD Medical School faculty. Maria Gomez is a 21-year-old Latina who has come to the doctor's office because of stomach pains that she has had for the past 2 days; a friend had told her it might be a bladder infection. Maria is a college student who has started work on her master's degree. She lives at home and is still covered by her parents' health insurance. She does not want her parents to know that she is sexually active or, if it comes up in the visit to the doctor, that she might be pregnant, or even that she is dating the boyfriend they disapprove of, because he is neither Latino nor Catholic.

---

[2] The patient's name, Maria Gomez, is a pseudonym. Certain other identifying characteristics of the real patient have also been changed to protect her identity. This is true not only for Maria Gomez but also for all the SP case examples in this book.

The Maria Gomez case materials in Appendix A consist of 11 documents, including the demographic form, the presenting situation and instructions to the student, the training materials, a printed computer version of the case checklist, the guide to the checklist, the guidelines for giving written feedback, the pelvic/rectal exam results, one version of an interstation exercise along with the interstation exercise key, as well as a separate case summary and an abridged checklist, both of which are intended for use by the candidates when auditioning for the part of this patient.[3]

In Appendix B are a number of sample documents you might find helpful in your own training of SPs. The SP Profile Form can be used to collect specific demographic information on each SP during auditioning. Once a candidate is selected, the sample Letter of Agreement can serve as a contract with the SPs to record their commitment to the SP training program. Although this document is not legally binding, it spells out the expectations you have of the SPs regarding training and actual exam administrations that they are required to participate in. Because it is advantageous to you and the SPs to video record all of their performances both during training and the actual exam administrations, you might want to have your SPs sign a Recorded Image Consent-and-Release Form, such as the one in Appendix B, before they begin training.

THE ROOTS OF OUR WORK

As you will see, I have made a strong connection in this book between the art of SP coaching, the dramatic arts, and the authenticity of our SPs' performances in the service of training future generations of physicians. The origins of drama and the art of acting are the subject of speculation among historians, anthropologists, and archeologists. However, it is reasonably certain that formal drama started in Greece, the birthplace of Western political thought, art, philosophy, and medicine (Geldard, 2000).

During the 5th century B.C.E., competitive drama festivals were state occasions and considered part holiday celebration, part religious ritual. Drama, as conceived by the major Greek tragedians, Aeschylus, Sophocles, and Euripides, was not merely for entertainment, but apparently was believed to have spiritual and healing potential by leading "the attentive listener through an emotional, intellectual, and spiritual. . . conflict, resulting in catharsis" (Geldard, 2000, p. 202). It is also clear that the cult of

---

[3] Note: In Appendix A, the Gomez documents have been kept in the order they are used as case materials by the coach and SP. For this reason, they are not numbered by order of appearance in the main text of the book.

Asklepios, the compassionate Greek god of healing, incorporated drama as well as worship, athletic events, and music into the care of its devotees' health and well-being. So we can see that since the inception of drama, acting and dramatic storytelling have been part of the art of medicine. It is humbling to realize that our work with standardized patients in medical education puts us in touch with such an ancient and noble history and gratifying to think that the arts of acting and medicine once again are being joined in the 21st century—this time to support the training of those whose work it will be to heal and ease the suffering of us all.

REFERENCES

Colliver, J. A., & Williams, R. G. (1993, June). Technical issues: Test application. *Academic Medicine, 68*(6), 454–460.

Geldard, R. G. (2000). *Ancient Greece: A guide to sacred places.* Wheaton, IL: Quest Books.

Petrusa, E. R. (2002). Clinical performance assessments. In G. R. Norman, C. P. M. Van der Vleuten, & D. I. Newble, (Eds.), *International handbook of research in medical education* (pp. 673–709). Dordrecht, The Netherlands: Kluwer Academic.

Coaching Standardized Patients

*For Use in the Assessment of
Clinical Competence*

PART ONE

Required Skill Sets: Developing the Expertise Needed to Coach Standardized Patients

CHAPTER ONE

Overview: The Art and Practice of Coaching Standardized Patients

The quality of any clinical skills examination using standardized patients depends on the coach's ability to guide well-chosen SPs to accurately and realistically portray the patient on whom the case is based and to accurately record what happened during a clinical encounter with each examinee. To competently do this work with standardized patients requires coaches to have certain kinds of expertise in a number of areas. Coaches must know and effectively use various training methods, techniques, and procedures to assist the SPs in accomplishing these goals. As professionals, SP coaches must have both the commitment and the coaching skills that it takes to assure that their SPs' performances and completed checklists meet the highest standards. We make this commitment so that the medical students have a fair and realistic opportunity to demonstrate their clinical skills and so that their scores accurately reflect their true level of competence.

Over the years within our discipline, a methodology has emerged to assure the coach's success in helping SPs meet the goals of performance and accuracy. But in addition to a methodology, there is an art to working with standardized patients—just as there is an art to working with real patients in the field of medicine. In our work with standardized patients, the methodology for training unites with the art of coaching—which relies on awareness, intuition, and the dramatic arts. It was my intent in writing this book that both the art of coaching and the practical aspects of training standardized patients would get the equal attention that each deserves.

As a coach, you may already have had experience working with standardized patients and are quite capable of training most of your SPs to give

3

factually accurate and convincing performances; in other words, performances that no one—faculty, medical students, yourself included—would challenge as being *un*realistic. Nonetheless, this book offers you specific ways to work with SPs so that you can elicit more deeply nuanced performances from them—performances that are so consistently believable that not only the medical students, but even you, forget that they are simulations.

THE COLLABORATION IN STANDARDIZED PATIENT WORK

No matter what we call this work with SPs—coaching, training, directing—at its best, it is a collaboration among the case author, the faculty, the SP coach, and the SPs. The success of this collaboration depends on

- having a well-written clinical case with well-defined objectives, including training materials with clear descriptions and medical details that are appropriately described for the SPs' use, along with enough "backstory" to at least hint at the complexity of the patient as a person;
- working effectively with SPs who have the natural or acquired facility to bring the patient to life, and
- continually developing our coaching abilities.

For those of you who are new to standardized patient training—whether you are a beginning or aspiring coach or simply an interested reader—I have briefly outlined the sequence of events in SP work, from developing the patient case to administering the exam and reporting the results. Although this process may vary from institution to institution, these are the common steps in preparing for and administering a clinical practice examination (CPX). Included are activities that generally follow the CPX once the performance data have been collected.

- After the decision is made to administer a CPX, a group of medical school faculty is convened to determine the objectives and what the exam is to assess; for example, which clinical skills, organ systems, types of clinical situations (chronic, acute, emergent, behavioral, grave diagnosis, etc.) should be represented.
- Guidelines are written to define for faculty authors the essential requirements for each case that will fulfill the assessment objectives of the exam.
- Faculty physicians are then asked to select from their clinical

practices real patients (who meet these requirements) to serve as anonymous models for the SP case development.

- A faculty physician (preferably the one whose patient is serving as the anonymous model) writes the case, in collaboration with the SP coach. (See Appendix A, Maria Gomez, for an example of a complete set of case materials.)
- The SP coach recruits candidates for each of the cases that have been written, then schedules a series of training sessions and a practice ("mock") exam with the SPs. (See Part Two for the training procedures and the Practice Exam protocols.)
- The actual CPX is administered for the number of days necessary to assess all of the medical students who are required to take the exam.
- A faculty committee (including the evaluator who analyzes the CPX data) determines pass/fail cuts.
- Students receive their CPX score reports and are informed whether they have passed or will need to participate in remediation, if they have failed.
- Remediation activities are planned for individual students based on their needs as identified by the CPX score reports.
- If students are required to pass the CPX in order to graduate from medical school, those needing remediation might be required to take and pass another CPX (which is different, but comparable to the original) to demonstrate that their skills meet the medical school's requirements.

THE UNIQUENESS OF STANDARDIZED PATIENT WORK

We and our SPs are co-creators of an imaginary world that needs to feel, smell, sound, and look as real as if it were the world of an actual patient being seen and treated by a practicing physician. As "artistic" members of the medical education team, our collective task as SP coaches is the manipulation of reality through the performances of our SPs to an important end: to provide experiential learning for medical students and performance assessment of their clinical competence. As coaches, we accomplish this task by communicating our understanding of who the patient is intellectually to the SPs and by guiding their performances with clear direction during their training. At the same time we must also be comfortable with giving the SPs the leeway to experiment with our expressed vision of the patient so that they too can contribute their talents to the unfolding of their performance as the patient with medical students in the simulated clinical setting.

The SPs' Performance Environment

The most obvious circumstance that makes standardized patient work unique is the environment in which the SPs give their performances—a hospital or clinical examination room. When standardized patients are used for medical students' clinical skills assessment, the SPs are not playing to an audience of students from a stage as they might be when they are incorporated into medical teaching demonstrations. SPs do not generally perform in an ensemble, although occasionally a given case might require more than one SP, such as in scenarios requiring a member of a standardized family to accompany another family member to the doctor for a check-up. Nor are the SPs primarily acting for a camera so that their work can be captured on video or film for entertainment or educational purposes. In the context in which our standardized patients are performing, they are playing the role of the patient in order to help medical school faculty assess the clinical competence of their medical students or residents.

The SPs' Improvisational Framework

SPs should be working from written training materials that provide them with a detailed description of the patient case or framework from which they can improvise responses to the medical student's inquiries, based in part on the student's interaction style. This framework might include specific lines that must be delivered exactly as written by the coach and the case author, but because the interaction between the medical student and the SP is by its nature improvisational, most of the framework is a narrative that includes all of the key information the SP needs in order to factually and consistently present an accurate portrayal of the patient, her medical problem, her emotional state, and her interaction style.

Now, here is the true uniqueness of what we do. Instead of being on stage or in a film studio repeating the fixed lines of a script, the SP is most often performing in a clinical exam room, face to face with one other person—the medical student (examinee)—who is also improvising within a defined framework during the clinical interaction. Each time the scenario unfolds encounter after encounter during the clinical exam, it will be both standardized[1] and unique. Both performers know the basic structure of the encounter, but only the SP knows the scenario—the story line of the patient case. Both are improvising, but the student doctor's task is to solve the problem the SP presents or to support the patient

---

[1] By standardized, I mean that each SP trained for this case will portray the same patient in such a consistent way that each medical student will be presented with the same challenge every time.

through the healing process, that is, to discover from her story and by examination what might be causing the patient's symptoms, or to work with her in other ways, such as helping the patient understand her illness, make necessary life style changes, deal with the grieving process, and so forth. This interaction of the SP with the medical student, in the name of clinical skills assessment and learning, is a most extraordinary happening.

SOME QUALITIES OF EFFECTIVE COACHES

Although there are many facets to being a standardized patient coach, the following are a few of the qualities and practices of those coaches who are regarded as truly expert. All skillful coaches need to:

Know Something About Acting and Directing

The task of coaching a standardized patient portrayal is ultimately about the SPs' performances and what the coach can do to help them shape the performances they are aiming for. Therefore, besides making sure that the SPs' performances are factually accurate, it is important for the coach to understand something about acting, because acting is what the SPs are doing. They are acting the part of a real patient whether they have formal training or not. It is even better if we have done some acting ourselves, or better yet, if we have been an SP. From such firsthand experience, we are better able to understand what the SPs are experiencing and better able to find ways to help them accomplish the common goals we are working toward. So, the more we know experientially about acting and directing (which can be acquired on the job while coaching)—as well as all the other performance challenges an SP has to deal with—the better coaches we will become. The beauty of this work is that there is always something to learn, always a more refined way to engage with our SPs. If we approach the work with this mindset, it will always be interesting and can provide a lifetime of discovery, both personal and professional. In short, standardized patient coaching can become for us the art that it truly is.

Develop Trusting Relationships With Their SPs

The relationship should be one of mutual respect, understanding, and love of the work—also trust. Because the director [coach] represents the eye which helps the actor [SP] to decide the form in which what he does will take place.
—Morris Carnovsky (as quoted in Funke & Booth, 1961, p. 285)

The director–actor relationship described by Carnovsky, one of the original actors of the Group Theatre, also aptly describes the ideal relationship of the SP coach and the SPs. It is the coach's vision of the patient case that enables the SPs to develop the "form" in which they will portray the patient. There are many ways for coaches and SPs to develop the kind of relationship that Carnovsky advocates, but I believe the key is to observe how you instinctively work as a coach so that you become aware of the style that is most natural for you. What ultimately works for you will be what you and your SPs are comfortable with. No matter what your style of interaction, it is your *awareness* of what you are doing that will keep you from either underestimating the SPs' capabilities and giving them directions for every nuance of their performances or, conversely, overestimating your actor–SPs' skills and putting them on a pedestal because you are not an actor and may feel uneasy directing them. When a coach operates out of this latter belief, the SPs usually get little or no direction whatsoever because the coach fears that his lack of knowledge will be found out. However, the truth is that establishing trust with the SPs and being up front and inviting them to let you know what they need from you (whenever they can) is a much more effective way to learn how to coach their portrayals.

Bring Enthusiasm and Sensitivity to Their Work

As directors of the SPs, we need to love the patient case and the process of bringing out in the SPs' performances the subtleties of the patient's personality and concerns. This enthusiasm can stimulate the imagination of the SPs, which is one of the key elements for bringing their portrayals to life. The danger is that some coaches can overdo their passion for the material and intimidate the SP to the point that he begins to question whether or not he can do what the coach is looking for. Therefore, the coach always needs to remain sensitive to the SPs' subtle cues—both verbal and nonverbal.

Carnovsky summarized nicely what many in acting believe is the director's job: to "illuminate" the material and "inspire the imagination" of the actors (Funke & Booth, 1961, p. 288). This can also be said for the SP coach. Illuminate and inspire!

Trust Their Intuition and What They Know

Perhaps at this point—especially if you are new to standardized patient work—you may be feeling a little overwhelmed. If so, it is helpful to remember that you actually know more about working with SPs than you might think you do. Just as good actors work out of their instincts, so will you. Trusting your intuition will do much to steer your work in the right direction. Above all, do not pretend to know something you do not. The SPs, more often than not, can sense a cover-up.

However, frequently apologizing for not knowing something will produce the same effect—loss of the respect you need in order to successfully guide the SPs through the training process. The trick is to learn what you can, then proceed respectfully with what you know. At the very least, you will always know more about the patient case, more about its challenges for the medical student, and more about the assessment objectives than the SPs, and—with preparation and study of the case materials—what you want from their performances. When you are stuck, get support and clarification from the SPs themselves, from health care professionals, from other SP coaches, and from books, workshops, and the Internet.

THE IMPORTANCE OF SELECTING THE RIGHT SPs

One of your roles as an SP coach is to find candidates who can perform the various patient cases for the Clinical Practice Examination. Chapter 5 provides extensive guidelines for recruiting the appropriate SPs, but here are a couple of other considerations regarding this aspect of your role as an SP coach. One consideration has to do with whether to hire actors or non-actors as SPs; the other, with finding the right SPs. If you can find SPs who fit the patient case you are casting, who can remember the facts and accurately fill out the checklist, and who can take direction—you will be able to focus more purposefully on coaching better performances from your SPs—primarily because you will not have to spend an inordinate amount of time monitoring and assisting them to maintain the high standards you want from them in all aspects of their performances.

Hiring Actors or Non-Actors as SPs

Should we hire actors or non-actors as SPs? Before I answer this important question, let me say that all SPs, whether they are actors or not, must possess certain characteristics. Every SP needs to be able to understand the training materials and, during their performance in an actual exam, exhibit an ability to concentrate on the medical students in order to observe their behaviors accurately and to respond to them appropriately. After their performance, the SPs must be able to remember what the medical student did and be literate enough to understand the import of all the patient case checklist items so that they can accurately record what transpired during the clinical encounter. If required, the SPs may also need to give feedback from the patient's perspective, either verbally to the student immediately after the encounter or in written comments that the students will receive later with their exam score report. These essential abilities have nothing to do with whether or not the chosen SPs have a background in acting.

Now, as to the actor/non-actor question—the short answer is—it depends. It depends on the kind of portrayal the case requires of the SP. These requirements fall on a continuum from cases that simply call for the SP to learn the facts and "play himself" to those that demand a consistent performance with specific emotional elements or complex psychological conditions. However, there are deeper issues underlying the beliefs and feelings about whether it is better to work with those who are naturally gifted, untrained performers (non-actors) or with those who have some formal training or experience in the theatrical arts (actors).

A large part of this actor/non-actor hiring decision depends on what we find when we audition our SP recruits for specific patient cases. Unless we make skillful choices in the SPs we select, we are likely to run into performance problems, whether the person has formal training in acting or not. In any event, this either–or dichotomy is an unnecessary concern, because the truth is that practical issues, more often than not, will win out. Sometimes a coach is simply forced by circumstances to work with whomever is available! Sometimes the coach is in a geographical area that is actor rich; at other times, it is more difficult to find someone trained in acting, even when the case demands such a person. So the best way to approach SP recruiting is to be open to working with both actors and non-actors alike.

Even if you do not work with professional actors as SPs or do not have any acting experience yourself, the language of what we do as coaches comes from the acting profession. SPs "play the part of" patients; medical students "act" or "pose as" doctors. Actors "train" in their profession. We "coach" or "direct" their performances. We have "auditions" or "casting calls." We do "call backs" when we cannot decide between two candidates. Then we "cast" the candidates who can best "perform" the patient cases. The SPs will be "improvising" within the framework of a "scenario" for the encounter, which is spelled out in the training materials. They will learn how to accurately and realistically "portray" the patient. The "role" of the patient not only includes the part of the patient's life that the medical student will experience directly in the clinical encounter, but also "character" information and "backstory" that will inform the SPs' performances and their understanding of the patient.

Eliciting Better Performances From Well-Chosen SPs

Underlying all of what I have said is the assumption that you are working with people who already have the skills and discipline to embrace your coaching and make it work in their performances of the particular patients you have chosen them to portray. In short, I assume that you have cast well, either by hiring non-actors who themselves have the physical qualities and temperament of the patient they will portray or by hiring actors who can take on those qualities.

Although it is not your job to specifically teach acting to your SPs, it *is* your job to help each SP understand the patient in the same way, as part of standardization, and to tweak performances that are already close to what you want. This is a significant part of what coaching is about. There is no time for us to teach acting to our SPs during training sessions, although we can certainly help talented SPs—actors or non-actors—come closer to the kind of performance we are looking for, by coaching them through any performance difficulties they might encounter. We do this by

- finding out what they are working with.
- offering suggestions (for how to work with the material).
- proposing one or another acting techniques for them to try.

You will find examples of these core coaching skills in this first part of the book, but I want to be clear that the focus of your training must, of necessity, operate from the assumption that from the very first training session, your SPs have both the capacity to give you what you are looking for and the ability to take direction.

If you have recruited, auditioned, and selected your standardized patients well, you will be working with the right people and your job will be what it is supposed to be—coaching the SPs to turn already acceptable portrayals into superb, subtly refined performances. This is the goal of the first part of this book: to shed light on how to get from your SPs skillful performances more in line with how you have imagined a particular patient to be.

THE SKILLS NEEDED TO BE AN SP

If you already have experience as a coach, you are most likely aware of the skills a person needs in order to be a standardized patient and how prominently these characteristics figure into SP selection. The skills fall into the following four distinct performance areas, all of which the SPs must carry out with exactitude.

The Ability to Portray a Patient

The SPs must be able to perform several aspects of a patient case. The most obvious is to learn the facts about the case and to give an accurate verbal history to the medical student during the clinical interview, which includes remembering the items on the case checklist so as not to volunteer information to the students inappropriately. In addition to what to say, the SPs must be able to determine exactly when and how much information to reveal to the student. They must also be able to realistically depict the patient's educational level, psychological state, and emotional condition, as well as to believably reproduce any abnormal physical findings that are part of the case.

For example, using the Maria Gomez patient case (see Appendix A), the SP needs to know the patient's family relationship and cultural background, be able to give specific details about her physical symptoms as well as simulate the appropriate level of pain during the physical exam, and to demonstrate this 21-year-old woman's fears and anxieties about the possibility of being pregnant.

The Ability to Observe the Medical Student's Behavior

At the same time that the SP is performing the case, she must be able to observe with precision the medical student's performance while they are interacting with one another. Some SPs are excellent actors, but get so involved in playing the part of the patient that they cannot simultaneously observe details regarding the clinical skills the medical student is performing during their encounter. Both capabilities are necessary to be a standardized patient.

For example, while portraying Maria Gomez and exhibiting her physical pain and psychological distress, the SP must at the same time note which parts of the case checklist the medical student is covering, while continually paying attention to how the student doctor is responding to Maria's other needs and concerns.

The Ability to Recall the Encounter and Complete the Checklist

Paired with the ability to observe what the medical student is doing, while performing the case, is the SP's ability to recall the details of the student's behavior immediately after the clinical encounter is finished. The ability to accurately complete the checklist is directly dependent on the SP's observation and flawless recall.

For example, once the clinical encounter has ended, the SP playing Maria Gomez must immediately fill out the checklist, recalling in detail what occurred between her and the medical student in all of the clinical skill areas being assessed.

The Ability to Give Feedback to the Student

In addition, the SP must be able to use all that she has observed in the encounter to give thoughtful, beneficial, and effective verbal or written feedback on the student's communication skills and interaction style from the point of view of the patient she was portraying.

For example, the SP must be able to write a description—from the perspective of Maria Gomez—of how she felt as the patient during the clinical encounter with the medical student.

With all these requirements, it is clear just how much is demanded and expected of the standardized patient. So much more is involved than initially meets the eye when watching an SP perform. Nevertheless, no matter how capable the SPs are, much of how well they do their job depends on the coach's ability to work with them.

THE SKILLS NEEDED TO BE AN SP COACH

In order to coach standardized patients to perform at the level of quality required in the assessment of medical students' clinical skills, SP coaches need to develop their abilities in three broad areas: (a) the basic set of clinical skills that every medical student needs to know, (b) some understanding of acting and acting techniques, along with (c) a few fundamental skills in directing to enhance the SPs' patient portrayals.

We need to know clinical skills both to coach the SPs in what to expect from the medical students they will be encountering and to coach them in how to respond to any and all actions taken by the student during a clinical exam. We also need to know these clinical skills in order to take on the role of medical students ourselves during our practice encounters with the SPs throughout their training.

In addition, we need to understand something about acting and directing in order to coach the kind of emotional/psychological performances called for in the case materials. This does not mean that we must have a background in medicine nor does it mean that we must have a background in acting to be able to coach SPs well. But it does mean that we need to learn a fair amount about clinical skills as well as acting and directing to adequately train our SPs to achieve the highest performance standards and the most realistic patient portrayals.

Therefore, in the next three chapters in Part One you will find information to help you grow in expertise if you need more knowledge or proficiency in any of these three basic coaching skill sets. Having said this, I want to be clear that the clinical skills chapter is not a course in how to diagnose and treat medical problems, but rather a guide for coaches to acquire and use the skills of medical history taking, physical examination, and patient–physician communication or interaction. Likewise, the chapter on acting is not a course in how to learn to act or how to teach SPs to act. Instead, it and the chapter on directing contain specific guidelines for working with and coaching persons who are either performers with a natural ability to reproduce the qualities of the patient you have hired them to portray or who are already skilled in the craft of acting.

These guidelines in the following chapters include ideas and suggestions, along with examples of basic skills and techniques that I have discovered over the past 20 years while working with standardized patients and other coaches and while conducting and participating in SP research. It is my hope that this information will support you in helping your SPs to shape their performances so that they are not only factually accurate and behaviorally authentic in their presentations and physical simulations, but utterly believable to the medical students who will work with them. With this in mind, what follows is a variety of offerings to support you in guiding your SPs toward the achievement of these goals in the simulated clinical encounter.

CHAPTER SUMMARY

This chapter on the art and practice of coaching standardized patients has

- provided an overview of standardized patient coaching;
- presented the sequence of events involving the collaboration of the medical school faculty, SP coaches, and SPs in creating and portraying the patient case and administering and scoring the CPX;
- described the uniqueness of standardized patient work both for the coach and the SPs, specifically the performance environment and improvisational nature of the SP patient portrayals;
- offered introductory guidelines for recruiting SPs (including working with actors and non-actors);
- depicted the role of the coach in helping the SPs to achieve performance and checklist accuracy, as well as in developing a mutual coach–SP relationship;
- enumerated the skills and abilities the SPs and the coach must bring to the work so that the SPs can give the most authentic performance of a patient case.

LOOKING AHEAD

The chapters in Part One are designed to support you in developing and refining your skills in the three broad areas that every SP coach needs: Chapter 2—Clinical Skills: Acquiring the Basic Doctoring Skills; Chapter 3—Acting: Understanding How the SPs Portray the Patient; and Chapter 4—Directing: Coaching to Deepen the SPs' Performances.

Clinical Skills: Acquiring the Basic Doctoring Skills

To assure that our standardized patients are performing at the level of quality required of them, coaches need to know something about the four basic clinical skill sets that are the foundation of every clinical encounter, whether that interaction is between a practicing physician and a real patient or between a medical student and a standardized patient. These four clinical skill sets include

- history taking.
- physical examination.
- patient–physician interaction or communication skills.
- information sharing or patient education.

LEARNING THE FOUR CLINICAL SKILL SETS

In this chapter, I describe some specific ways to acquire enough understanding and expertise in the four clinical skill areas so that you can effectively train your SPs to handle any eventuality that might arise when they are working with the medical students.

History Taking

If you are coming to SP work without a background in medicine, before you can train the SPs to respond appropriately to the many ways that medical students approach a patient, it is important to learn how to take a complete medical history and how to interview a patient.

You can always start your training by using the items on the case checklist itself (see Appendix A4, Checklist) and supplementing them with other information contained in the training materials (see Appendix A3,

Training Materials), but you cannot rely solely on these items or you will end up skewing the training in the direction of items that only exist in these case materials. This will not adequately prepare the SPs for what they will encounter when working with the students. Therefore, as a first step in learning how to train your SPs, it will serve you well to acquire some basic, generic clinical skills, starting with history taking. There are a number of resources to help you do this. Here are a few:

Get the Syllabi From the Clinical Skills Courses Taught in Years I and II of Your Medical School Curriculum

Different institutions teach these basic clinical skills courses under various names. Look for the courses that include medical history taking, interviewing, and physical examination skills. Regardless of whether you use the manuals for these courses in your own skill development, reading them can help you discover what the medical students are learning and at what point in their training they are being taught these skills at your medical school.

Study the Same Texts That the Medical Students Use to Learn These Skills

Besides looking at the required textbooks being used at your institution, look for other books that are available on medical interviewing and history taking. You might find these two helpful:

- *The Complete Patient History* by Maurice Kraytman (1991). This book covers the sequential steps in history taking, discusses common unforeseen technical and psychological traps, and explains how to take a problem-solving approach to various patient symptoms and concerns. Most of the book is divided into specific organ–system symptoms with examples of questions to ask that systematically cover all the areas that are pertinent to that particular problem.
- *Sapira's Art and Science of Bedside Diagnosis* by Jane Orient and Joseph Sapira (2005). Although this text is primarily devoted to physical diagnosis, several excellent chapters at the beginning are devoted to the interview, the history, and the case record.

Get History Intake Forms From Clinics Associated With Your Medical School

Most primary care clinics have forms that patients are expected to fill out before seeing the doctor. These forms usually consist of questions that can be excellent resources for you as an SP coach. Most of the cases you will be developing and training are likely to be primary care-oriented; therefore, the best locations to find such forms would be internal medicine, family medicine, obstetrics-gynecology, geriatric medicine, pediatric, and adolescent medicine clinics.

Avail Yourself of Pharmaceutical Materials Designed for Patients

Drug companies often have excellent, informative booklets for consumers, encouraging them to ask themselves important questions regarding their symptoms and suggesting appropriate questions to ask their doctors. With a little adaptation, these questions can be incorporated into your own repertoire of questions that are appropriate for a specific disease or set of patient symptoms. All pharmaceutical companies have Web sites and are more than willing to share this kind of information with consumers.

Check With Associations and Societies Dedicated to a Specific Illness

Examples include the American Chronic Pain Association, the Arthritis Foundation, the National Lung and Heart Association, the American Cancer Society, the AARP, the Alzheimer's Association, among many others. As you learn more about the illnesses that you are training your SPs to portray, these organizations can be excellent sources of information and guidance regarding the origins, causes, symptoms, and other specifics of diseases, as well as possible treatment and prognosis. The more you know about the illness you are training the SPs to convey, the easier it will be to build a repertoire of questions that are appropriate to ask the patient when you are playing the role of the medical student during the SPs' training. This will make your work with the SPs more effective and realistic, precisely because of the breadth of understanding you incorporate into their training.

Physical Examination

In addition to history taking, most CPX cases require the medical students to perform a physical examination (PE) on the standardized patient. This means that the coach must be able to perform all the required physical exam maneuvers on the checklist in order to give the SPs practice in performing the simulated findings and in accurately filling out the physical exam portion of the checklist. The coach must be able to perform all maneuvers correctly and in variously incorrect ways—as well as any other physical exam maneuvers (not on the checklist) that the students are likely to perform in the clinical encounter.

Whenever an SP is required to reproduce a physical finding or a physical manifestation of a symptom or a medical or mental condition, our first order of business as a coach is

- to discover the external manifestations of the condition; for example, a person who has had a stroke might have paralysis in various parts of the body, including the limbs and face, and might only be able to speak in a slurred fashion, or might be unable to speak at all.
- to determine if there is an emotional or psychological component to the symptoms.
- to help the SPs understand the manifestations they must reproduce.
- to provide enough opportunities for the SPs to practice the manifestations—or the absence of normal responses—until they become so automatic that the SPs barely have to consciously think about producing these abnormal effects while performing the case.

These aspects of training require the coach to have (or acquire) some medical and clinical understanding. Therefore, in order to train SPs to produce simulated physical findings, you need to know something about the following three areas:

1. *Not only which physical findings the SP needs to simulate, but also how to reproduce those findings at will.* As coaches we must know exactly what needs to be physically simulated and precisely how the SP needs to produce those simulated findings. Howard Barrows (1999), the physician who first used standardized patients and the person responsible for the extraordinary growth of this methodology, has written an indispensable handbook on how to simulate physical findings, entitled *Training Standardized Patients to Have Physical Findings.*
2. *How to coach the SPs into authentically reproducing the required physical simulations.* The first step in coaching this aspect of a performance involves demonstrating to the SPs what the simulated physical findings look like. Then as each SP tries to reproduce these findings, our job is the relentless pursuit of detail as we give almost simultaneous feedback to the SP who is "trying on" the simulated physical responses for the first time. This aspect of coaching the SP is similar to coaching an athlete or a dancer. For example: If you were talking an SP through how she is to hold herself when

she moves with a particular kind of back pain in a sitting position, it might sound something like this excerpt from a transcript of an actual coaching session:

> Good, you're holding yourself off-center, favoring the side with the pain, but as you answer my questions, you're moving too many other parts of your body separately. Hold your back up straight and move your body all of a piece as if you were wearing a straight jacket. Remember, you feel the pain even when you try to change positions in the chair. Place your arms on the chair to help make the position change. That's good! You can even use your arms to raise your entire body off of the chair and get yourself on the edge of the seat before you try to stand up. Can you feel that? That's it. Now, you've got it.

3. *How to do whatever the student might be expected to do.* In preparing to train the SPs on a given case, we must first acquire an understanding of the physical exam maneuvers involved, then learn how to perform them correctly ourselves. We also need to know which other parts of the physical examination the students are likely to perform even though they might not be tested on those maneuvers. We must learn how to do this with dexterity so that we can vary how we perform the physical examination during training. Performing the maneuvers correctly with ease ourselves is important in order to give the SPs adequate practice in producing the physical simulations required and to train them to assess the quality of the maneuvers being done on them when they are filling out the checklists on the students' performances.

Here are a few ways you can acquire the necessary background before learning to perform any of the specific physical exam skills required by a given case:

Study Textbooks

Look up the maneuvers in the physical examination teaching text that the students in your institution are using. Three of the more commonly used texts are

- *Bates' Guide to Physical Examination and History Taking* by Lynn Bickley and Peter Szilagyi (2003).
- *Mosby's Guide to Physical Examination* by Henry Seidel et al. (2003).
- *Textbook of Physical Diagnosis: History and Examination* by Mark Swartz (2002).

If you are not a health care professional and, thus, have no experience performing physical examinations, this part of SP coaching might seem daunting. Therefore, I suggest that you learn how to perform the physical examination maneuvers as required in each case you are about to train, rather than try to learn the overall details of the complete physical examination all at once, up front. The reason I suggest this is that you will likely forget details of various parts of the physical examination if you do not use them immediately and regularly. It is more efficacious to learn what you need to know as it arises on a case-by-case basis.

Study Video Recordings of Physical Examination Demonstrations

Go on the Internet or to the medical library and watch video recordings of the particular part of the physical exam you need to learn. This will familiarize you with what the examination maneuvers look like in action while they are being performed. Some textbooks have companion DVDs that demonstrate in real time the performance of the physical exam maneuvers. Better yet, find out what the students at your medical school are using as teaching materials because they are learning the same maneuvers you want to acquire.

Practice. Practice. Practice.

Go over the physical maneuvers that you have observed and studied on anyone who will work with you—a friend, your partner, a colleague— anyone who is willing to let you practice hands on what you have conceptually learned about the physical examination.

Learn Which Physical Findings Can Be Simulated

Of the kinds of physical findings that can be simulated, the most obvious include

- physical sensations or loss of sensation (pain, tingling, numbness).
- increased reflexes, weakness, change in gait (stumbling, limping).
- dizziness, vertigo.

In addition, a number of not-so-obvious physical conditions can be simulated quite realistically. The most valuable resource on how to reproduce external physical signs is Barrow's aforementioned handbook. In it you will find practical descriptions on how to teach your SPs to produce more than 50 physical manifestations of various medical conditions, including different ways that pain presents physically, as well as such seemingly impossible-to-simulate conditions as coma, various complex neurological conditions like Parkinson's Disease, lid lag for hyperthyroidism, pneumothorax (collapsed lung on one side of the chest in which no breath sounds can be heard), carotid bruits (the sound created by a blockage of blood flow in the artery of the neck going to the brain), blindness, hyperventilation (without the SP getting dizzy), and various levels of muscle weakness. Barrow's handbook should be in the library of everyone who is coaching standardized patients.

There are other ways to simulate physical conditions:

- *Using equipment that is rigged.* Sometimes the simulation can be handled by altering the medical equipment, such as changing the readings on the sphygmomanometer to simulate high blood pressure.
- *Using make-up and moulage.* Other conditions (for example, jaundice, bruises, moles, and other skin conditions) can be imitated by the use of special make-up. More complicated wounds can be simulated by the use of moulage (the molding and crafting of various types of plastic, along with paint and make-up, to simulate different kinds of lacerations). If you can locate a center where first responders do practice runs for disaster preparedness, you will likely find moulage artists who create very realistic wounds on simulated disaster victims. When you need this kind of simulation, these moulage artists might be willing to work with you—or teach you how—to create the more complex kinds of simulated wounds you require.

Use Authentic Alternative Methods When a Physical Finding Cannot Be Simulated

Even with all these simulation possibilities, there are certain physical findings that still cannot be simulated, such as heart murmurs, enlarged livers, or pupils that do not constrict when light is shined in the eyes. To circumvent these challenges, a number of medical schools have made it standard practice to have the SP give the student this information by other, more or less valid means. However, these methods (some more than others) disrupt the realism of the encounter by requiring the SP to give information that is out of character for the patient they are portraying.

Of these less skillful methods, the least obtrusive to case authenticity is to instruct the medical student not to perform certain parts of the overall physical exam (for example, the more intimate kinds of examinations—rectal, genital, pelvic, or breast), but to simply say to the SP at the appropriate point in the physical, that he would like to do a rectal exam, for example. In response, the standardized patient, as trained, indicates where in the clinic exam room the student can find the results for that particular part of the examination.

The two other most commonly used methods are more disruptive of the reality of the student–SP interaction during the clinical encounter. They both involve abnormal physical exam findings that cannot be simulated. In one scenario, the SP hands the medical student a written description of the abnormal physical findings *as* the student attempts to perform that exam maneuver. In the other scenario, *after* the student has completed the PE maneuver, the SP breaks character to tell the student to disregard what he has heard, felt, or seen, and assume that he has experienced something else. These methods should be avoided because they harm the simulation in varying degrees by breaking the illusion of reality hard won by the careful training and performance of the standardized patients.

There are a couple of ways around these contrived methods. One is to write only cases for which you are reasonably certain you can recruit SPs who actually have the real physical findings the case requires, or to write cases, as much as possible, with physical findings that *can* be simulated. This is not as great a limitation as it might seem at first. By using Barrows' suggestions—along with your own and your faculty's creative ideas—you can provide realistic simulation alternatives that once seemed inconceivable.

Another option is to use the post-encounter write-ups to open up the diagnostic possibilities of the case. You can have the students listen to abnormal heart sounds, see abnormal retinal images, get abnormal lab results, and so on; then ask them how these new findings have changed their thinking regarding the differential on the patient. This use of post-encounter exercises has the added potential of teasing out the students' clinical reasoning and at the same time maintaining the authenticity of the actual clinical encounter.

Acquire Proficiency in Performing the Physical Exam

Once you understand specifically what the physical exam entails, can visualize the examination techniques, and have had a little practice with these maneuvers, you are ready to acquire the proficiency you need in order to train your SPs to respond appropriately to any physical exam maneuvers that might be performed on them. The following methods—beginning with the most effective—will help you develop this proficiency so that you can train your SPs with skill and confidence:

1. *Request that a health care professional be identified as coresponsible for the training of the SPs in the physical examination.* Getting a health care professional (such as a faculty physician, nurse, or physician's assistant) to be the clinician responsible for supporting you in training the SPs is not always easy, but, if you are new to this field, it is worth the effort.

   Sometimes such a clinician is the person responsible for your high-stakes clinical skills examination. Other times, your clinician partner might be someone who wants to develop a case for use in a particular clerkship. As you work through the best way to get the support you need, do not feel intimidated by not knowing how to do the training for the physical examination. If you are not a clinician, no one should expect you to know anything about this area. At the same time, do feel confident that with practice and observation of your skills by a clinician, you will eventually learn how to do these maneuvers—at least as well as the students do them.

   If you are training for a clinical examination, you should be working with both a checklist and a guide to the checklist (see Appendix A5, Guide to the Checklist). Not only can the checklist and the guide serve as outlines for the clinician to teach you and/or your SPs, but they can also serve as blueprints for your learning of the physical exam components and for coaching the SPs in them.

2. *Find someone to guide you in learning how to do the physical examination and to verify the accuracy of the simulations.* If you cannot get a designated clinician to participate in the training of your SPs, the next best approach to the training of physical findings is to have a clinician teach you how to do what is necessary before you work with your SPs. The most efficient way to do this is to simply set up a session in which the clinician trains you to do the physical examination on one other person.

   This one-on-one training should consist not only of your watching the clinician perform the physical exam maneuvers on another person but also of your performing the same maneuvers on the other person while the clinician observes you. Thus, the clinician can reinforce, as well as correct, what you are doing. I suggest video recording the session so that you can review specifics as you practice the physical exam procedures in preparation for working with the SPs.

3. *Sit in on sessions when the medical students are being taught physical exam techniques.* It is very helpful to learn how to do the physical exam while the students are learning to perform the same skills. This will give you the advantage of knowing what and how the students are being taught to perform the maneuvers that your SPs are going to be rating.

4. *Take standardized patient training workshops.* A number of workshops are given throughout the country and at conferences planned by our professional organization, the Association of Standardized Patient Educators (www.aspeducators.org). Another excellent general resource for connecting with other SP educators and finding out about local and regional workshops is the SP Trainers' Mailing List (http://depts.washington.edu/hsasf/clinical/sp.html). Many of these workshops include training procedures as well as demonstrations on how to train various simulated physical findings, and how to use make-up and moulage to enhance SP simulations.

5. *Get information from other sources.* Always keep your eye open for ways to get the latest guidelines on physical examination procedures; for example, the American Cancer Institute Guidelines on the Breast Exam or the set of physical examination cards published by the Association of American Medical Colleges (1999). These cards spell out the documentation requirements that must be used to substantiate a beneficiary charge to Medicare. As you might guess, the set of criteria listed in these cards is thorough and extensive. It is helpful to have such a resource handy for your own learning and for case development as well.

6. *Always have a clinician check out the work you have done with your SPs.* No matter how experienced you become as a coach—or even if you, the SP coach, are a clinician yourself—it is a good idea to have someone else take a look at your work with the SPs lest you have inadvertently overlooked something. This clinician verification is built into Training Session Four (see chapter 10, The First Dress Rehearsal).

Patient–Physician Interaction (PPI)/Communication Skills

Another set of skills the coach needs to have in order to train SPs to observe and assess medical students is clinical communication skills. Patient–physician interaction encompasses a set of skills that have been proven "to enhance health outcomes" (Bayer Institute for Health Care Communication,[1] 2003, p. 3). In addition, physicians possessing these skills enrich the therapeutic relationship by creating an atmosphere in which patients trust that the physician is not only medically competent and has integrity but also genuinely cares about them as people, their psychological experience of the illness, and their overall well-being. In such a relationship, patients also feel safe enough to share not only their

---

[1] Now known as the Institute for Healthcare Communication (www.healthcarecomm.org).

symptoms but also their worries and ideas about what might be causing these symptoms.

In 2001, a group of leading experts in the field of health care communication convened to "facilitate the development, implementation and evaluation of communication-oriented curricula in medical education," which produced the The Kalamazoo Consensus Statement ("Essential Elements," 2001, p. 390). This group, which included a number of prominent researchers who had developed individual communication models, focused their attention on "identifying specific communication tasks" essential to effective physician–patient interactions (Kalamazoo, p. 391). The idea was to designate tangible competencies and skills that could be taught and evaluated. What these experts produced was published as "The Kalamazoo Consensus Statement," a list of evidence-based core communication competencies and standards, laid out simply and clearly, by which communication skills can be measured. For our purposes, as SP coaches, the spelling out of these core competencies is invaluable for designing communication checklists and for training SPs to assess the PPI items (see Appendix A4, Checklist and Appendix A5, Guide to the Checklist). The Kalamazoo Consensus Statement outlined these seven core competencies:

1. Build a relationship.
2. Open the discussion.
3. Gather information.
4. Understand the patient's perspective.
5. Share information.
6. Reach agreement on problems and plans.
7. Provide closure. (p. 391)

For you as an SP coach, these core competencies can serve as a framework to learn the specific communication skills you want to incorporate into your training encounters. However, more than technical expertise is needed to ensure a successful, therapeutic connection between a physician and the patient. That extra something has to do with the *manner* in which the communication skills come across to the patient. For the medical student to be effective, he must possess, develop, or adapt his style to ensure that the techniques he is using come across in the caring, respectful manner he intends. For you to be effective as a coach, you must be able to mix and match different communication competencies with a variety of interaction styles that represent the level and diversity of students the SPs will be working with. The best way to learn to portray a variety of student styles is to carefully watch them interacting with real or simulated patients while you make notes on the specifics things the students do that contribute to how they are coming across.

The SPs must learn to identify the specific communication skills the medical students are using and how their style of delivery is impacting their effectiveness in creating that therapeutic bond with the patient that the SPs are portraying. The best way to train SPs to understand the Patient–Physician Interaction scale, by which they rate the students on the checklist, is by having them *use* it. Both a common intellectual understanding of the items and the SPs' judgment are integral to their training to use the PPI scale. As an intrinsic outgrowth of this training, the SPs learn what is reasonable to expect regarding how a patient should be treated by a physician. The natural tendency of most untrained SPs, no matter how specific the communication items are, is to rate all of them according to whether or not they liked the student or according to their style of interaction. In other words, if coaches are not watchful, the SPs might turn the PPI into an assessment of the student's *niceness*. To overcome this halo effect, you must give the SPs plenty of practice with plenty of variety so that they can learn to assess the student's interaction skills with each PPI item, without letting their like or dislike of the student unduly influence their ratings of the student's communication skills.

Interpreting the medical student's behavior when filling out the PPI is a different kind of task for the SPs than any of the others. The subtleties of understanding the import of what you will be asking of the SPs are sometimes lost on them until they are actually filling out the checklist after the clinical encounter. What you will be asking of the SPs is that they rate the student by filling out the PPI from the patient's perspective without forgetting what they—the ones performing the case—have learned about effective communication skills.

Another difference between the PPI and all the other items on the checklist is that the history, physical exam, and information-sharing items are rated on a dichotomous (yes/no; done/not done) scale, whereas the PPI items are rated on a Likert (continuum) scale. So the SPs must not only understand the intent behind each of the PPI items, but must also know how the items are anchored on the continuum. For example, on a scale of 1 to 6 (where 1 = Outstanding, 2 = Very Good, 3 = Good, 4 = Marginal, 5 = Needs Improvement, 6 = Unacceptable), how is the SP to mark a student on the "established personal rapport" item, which is defined in part in the guide to the checklist as, "Showed interest in me as a 'person,' not just in my condition"? Is it enough for the SP to give the medical student a "very good" if he seemed to be interested in what the patient had to say but did not ask anything about the patient's life, job, or family, or did not follow up on any of the patient's clues about his concerns?

It is only by actually using the PPI scale with the individual items while assessing the students' behaviors that the SPs will begin to really grasp the meaning of the items and the level of communication quality that is designated by each increment on the rating scale. Remember it is not necessary for you and the SPs to have 100% agreement on all items on a Likert-type scale, but you should aim to be within one number/one increment of each other, with each SP being able to recount specific student behaviors that caused her to rate each item as she did.

A coach who is grounded in PPI skills can then teach the SPs how to respond to different medical student approaches by combining various communication skills and styles during the practice encounters. The following are examples of some of the ways these skills and styles might be combined.

Finding Out the Patient's Perspective and Addressing the Patient's Feelings

In the following example, the coach is playing a student who knows he needs to find out how the patient perceives what is going on and address the patient's feelings, but the coach intentionally makes a common student mistake when the patient does not respond as he would like:

> Let's say, as the student in the practice encounter you are working at building rapport with the patient that the SP is portraying in order to gain the patient's trust. Early in the encounter, you suspect that the patient is reticent about something. (Of course, as the coach, you know the patient is reticent about something because you know what is in the training materials.) So you decide to use the technique of reflecting back to the patient what you are sensing—however, you choose to say rather abruptly and in a dispassionate tone of voice exactly what is on your mind: "You seem reluctant to tell me something. You don't need to hold anything back." Although the patient does have something on his mind, because of the manner of delivery, the patient feels accosted and so correctly denies his truth by saying, "I'm not holding back on anything."
>
> To challenge the SP further, you pursue the patient with "You *need* to tell me what's on your mind if I'm going to be able to help you." And with that tone, that choice of language, whatever rapport had been established up to that point has likely been destroyed. Now, as coach-playing-medical student, you can decide whether to simply ignore the situation (and hope it goes away as many students do) or try to rebuild rapport as the practice encounter continues.

Just looking at this small segment from a training interview, you can see the kinds of choices and judgment calls the coach-as-student needs to make to prompt the SP to give responses based on both *what* the coach said and *how* the coach said it. The coach's portrayal of the medical student's lack of skill includes the use of awkward language, the abrupt in-your-face observation to the patient, then the attempt to force the patient to give information he does not have or does not want to reveal yet. Thus the coach has given the SP the opportunity to decide not only how to respond in the encounter but also how to rate the student on the PPI items having to do with building rapport and understanding the patient's perspective.

Using Open-Ended Questions

The verbal or nonverbal encouragements from the student, which allow the patient to share what's on his or her mind, can come in the form of open-ended questions like these:

- "Can you tell me more about ... ?"
- "Anything else you are concerned about?"
- "Any other symptoms you've been experiencing?"
- "Anything else you think we should address in this visit today?"

The students are taught to focus on these kinds of questions at the beginning of their clinical encounters, but they may choose to ask them at other times as well. Open-ended questions are meant to encourage patients to share with the physician what they have been experiencing physically and how they have been feeling emotionally. Defining for the SPs the guidelines they are to follow for disclosing information is essential when coaching the SPs on how to deal with any appropriately asked open-ended question (see Appendix A3, Training Materials, and A5, Guide to the Checklist). These guidelines should include the following:

- Under what specific circumstances to give information to the student.
- What that information should consist of.
- The order in which the SP is to reveal the information.
- How many bits of information are to be given for a single question (or invitation).

These disclosure guidelines are crucial in training the SPs to be able to give impeccable performances. Note that these guidelines are multileveled. It is your responsibility as an SP coach to lead the SPs to understand this layering of information and then to coach their performances so that they accurately reflect the case author's intentions. If guidelines such as these do not exist in the case materials you are working with, you will need to create them before you start training your SPs. Here is a simple example that takes into consideration the first two disclosure guidelines:

Let's say that the patient has told the doctor that the reason for her visit is to get a check-up, but, like many patients who come in for check-ups on an irregular basis, she doesn't reveal everything she is worried about in her opening statement. If the student doctor asks any appropriate open-ended question such as "Are you worried about anything in particular?" or "Anything else on your mind?", the case materials might direct the patient to offer this response: "Well, my sister was just diagnosed with breast cancer—so I've been a little concerned about that."

Coaching open-ended questions in a clinical skills assessment can seem like a complex task, especially if you or any of your SPs are new to this aspect of training. In truth, it *is* a more advanced skill to address, because it requires higher-order thinking and judgment on the part of the SPs. There is no denying that this type of training does take extra effort, but it is worth it because the outcome—with the SPs being able to more realistically and effectively reinforce and assess the students' communication skills—is closer to how we are training our students to interact.

Asking Compound Questions

To save time, students often acquire the unskillful habit of asking a string of questions in one query to the patient. These compound questions come in many varieties, for example: "Do you have diabetes, high blood pressure, cardiovascular disease, high cholesterol, problems with your liver ...?" or this example which is taken from an actual exam: "So what's your lifestyle like—are you health conscious, do you watch your diet and exercise, or do you drink alcohol or smoke, or do anything like that?" This assailing of the patient with a string of questions is something we want the students to become aware of because most patients cannot keep track of what they are being asked if they are not given the chance to answer the items one by one. The students are often unaware of how little time it takes to give the patient a moment to answer each query, if asked one at a time. Equally important is the fact that asking a list of questions in tandem, without a pause, can provide a cover for the patient who is inclined to hide something the student has just asked about, such as the use of alcohol, tobacco, or drugs.

To help the student modify this style of questioning, consider having the SPs only answer the last query in a long list. Using the previous examples, the SP would respond. "No, I don't have any problems with my liver ... " or "I used to smoke, but I quit a few years ago." However you decide to train the SPs to answer multiple questions strung together, they should make explicit what their reply refers to and not simply answer "yes" or "no" to a string of inquiries.

For more information on what we know from the research that has been done on communication skills in the medical setting, you can start with these two excellent resources:

- *Contemporary Issues in Medicine: Communication in Medicine,* Report III, Medical School Objectives Project (Association of American Medical Colleges, 1999).
- *The Annotated Bibliography for Clinician Patient Communication to Enhance Health Outcomes* by Maysel Kemp White and Kathleen Bonvicini (2003; see also www.healthcarecomm.com, Annotated Bibliographies). This bibliography is on the Web site of the Institute for Healthcare Communication (the former Bayer Institute for Health Care Communication).

Information Sharing (IS)/Patient Education Skills

In addition to being able to take a medical history, perform the requisite physical examination maneuvers, and employ various communication techniques in the training of our SPs, coaches must also learn to simulate different kinds of medical students as they educate the patients and/or share information with them about (a) what might be going on with them, (b) necessary follow-up care, (c) lifestyle changes the patient might need to make, and (d) any other relevant information the patient needs to know or that the training materials require the patient to ask. Once again, we have to do this by using different styles of student interaction and by purposefully including and excluding different information each time we practice with the SPs. This gives them a chance to master their responses to the students, and to determine in practice how and when to give those responses appropriately.

If the training materials you are working with do not include enough specific content about the information sharing/patient education part of the encounter, you can find such information for your training through the many resources that are now readily available on the Internet. Once again, associations devoted to specific illnesses have a wealth of information on their Web sites to help patients understand the disease, its management, treatment, and so on. Other training aids that SP educators find useful include medical references designed specifically for lay persons, such as those published by such reputable institutions as Johns Hopkins University, the National Library of Medicine, the Mayo Clinic, the Berkeley School of Public Health, or brochures and other printed materials available through physicians' offices.

The Connection Between Information Sharing and PPI Skills

Being able to proficiently share information and educate the patient are essential clinical communication skills that strengthen the physician's ability to influence and improve health outcomes in their patients. Besides knowing the relevant medical content, the student—or the coach when playing the medical student—must be able to demonstrate mastery of these skills by effectively connecting with the patient (SP) and by specifically addressing the patient's concerns. In other words, during the clinical encounter, at a minimum, the medical student must (a) determine what information is medically necessary to go over with the patient (SP), and (b) address whatever expressed or unexpressed needs the patient has. The student must then be able to offer that information, in a manner—and using language—the SP can understand, while exploring if the patient is truly comprehending what is being said. In short, what this means is that the student must interact meaningfully with the SP, not just deliver a lecture!

Once again, our creative challenge is to simulate a variety of student communication styles when we are running through practice encounters with our SPs. These styles can run the gamut from delivering a monologue/lecture (leaving little opportunity for the patient to participate) to an exchange of ideas, a conversation, or a negotiation with the patient, leading to a mutually agreeable plan of action at the end of the encounter. Your ability to perform accordingly relies on your knowledge and process skills, on your understanding of the content of the medical information, and on how adept you are at conveying that information differently from practice encounter to practice encounter.

To give the SPs adequate training in dealing with what is involved in a medical student's sharing of information with the patient, you need to know and have some technical mastery of these skills yourself. You also need to have some idea of what the students might suspect is going on with the patient, namely, content knowledge in the form of a differential diagnosis. Once you know the differential, you can look up information on the specific illnesses and/or have faculty share information you can use in training the patients.

In one practice encounter with the SPs, you might share information clearly and concisely in language the patient can understand. In other encounters, you might choose to give the SPs practice in dealing with a medical student who provides the patient with too much, or inappropriate, information for the circumstances. In other words, in the role of the medical student, you might deliberately

- overload the SP with information about heart disease or with detailed explanations of procedures that "might" have to be performed, or possible treatments, when all the patient really wants/needs to know is whether or not he has had a heart attack and what the next step in his care will be.

- counsel the SP to stop smoking and make other lifestyle changes that would be more appropriately dealt with at another visit because all the patient wants to know at this visit is whether he has a life-threatening illness because he has been coughing up blood.

Guidelines for What SPs Can/Cannot Do During Information Sharing

In terms of coaching the SPs how to perform when the student is sharing information or educating the patient, the coach and the SPs need to make certain decisions together. Here is an example of a relatively simple situation, but one that can cause problems if certain parameters are not explicitly addressed:

> Let's say the student is unclear in giving explanations or instructions to the patient. Should the SP be allowed to ask the student to clarify what she means? In determining whether to allow the SP to ask for clarification, one consideration is whether this action will confound any of the checklist items by leading the student into behaviors he should have displayed without prompting from the SP.

In this scenario, depending on the student behavior you want to assess, you might

- coach the SPs to not ask any clarifying questions and simply listen to whatever the student says.
- let the SPs ask for clarification but within limits, allowing them, for instance, to ask no more than two questions.
- require the SPs to wait to ask for clarification until the student prompts the SP by specifically inviting the patient to ask questions.

Sometimes restricting the SPs in this manner can frustrate them because it feels unnatural not to be able to ask a question when something is unclear or because the SPs want the students to know that their descriptions and explanations are bewildering to them. One way to alleviate these kinds of SP concerns is to provide an opportunity for them to give feedback to the students in the form of written comments that are part of the checklist. (For suggestions on how to coach SPs to give written feedback, see chapter 9.)

PORTRAYING THE MEDICAL STUDENT WITH THE SPs

Coaches need to be able to do most of the things that medical students are learning to do to become doctors because we must take on the role of the medical student when practicing clinical encounters with our SPs during their training. In addition, we must be able to portray medical students with diverse qualities, styles, and varying degrees of expertise.

When you first try to portray someone other than yourself, it might feel awkward. Sometimes coaches try to get over that discomfort by blatantly playing a bad student (usually not all that difficult when you are first starting to train!). The first rule of thumb is not to be seduced by the tendency to go to extremes. Do not portray anyone as too excessive or too overblown. This will not serve you or the SPs—because, in fact, your worst student imaginable does not exist. These kinds of training encounters usually end up being so bad that they do not give the SPs realistic practice, nor do they give them practical experience in remembering checklist details because the SPs often end up correctly filling out the checklist with all "no" and/or "not done" ratings.

The other precept is to only enact student qualities that will affect SPs' choices in performing the particular patient they are portraying, such as asking about specific issues that are in the training materials but not on the checklist; mixing up the order of the physical examination maneuvers in ways that students might realistically perform them so that the SPs sharpen their ability to produce the required simulations on command; giving the patient bad news at various places in the encounter (at the beginning, middle, or end), and so on.

The first time the SPs play the case with you, perform the interview with them in as thorough and as sensitive a manner as possible, covering a wide range of issues in the training materials and the checklist, using as skillful a communication style as you can. The first training interaction should not create too many challenges for the SPs, because this is the time for them to get a sense of how it feels to take on the characteristics of the patient during a full encounter. The importance of this strategy lies in building the SPs' confidence in the roles they are playing and in giving you an opportunity to sense where there might be some issues you need to address before giving them more advanced challenges.

Once the SPs have had a chance to get their feet wet and have gotten feedback from you on their portrayals, you can begin to add more complicated elements to the interviews. You can portray a student with less effective interaction skills, for instance, by not asking questions in a logical, organized way, by not asking any open-ended questions, or by not finding out the patient's perspective on his symptoms. You can portray students with behaviors that detract from their ability to connect with the patient by speeding through a number of medical questions and not letting the patient finish what he is saying, or by burying your face in the notes you are taking on your clipboard, and so on.

If there is one overarching principle to keep in mind when you are preparing the SPs for performance, it is this: *Mix it up*. Mix up everything that you do so that the SPs do not get used to a particular pattern in the unfolding of the practice encounters.

- Ask questions
  - that are not on the checklist as well as those that are.
  - in a different order each time you practice with the SPs.
  - in different ways (e.g., politely, coldly, disinterestedly, shyly, rapidly, without confidence, in an organized or disorganized manner, etc.).
  - using language that is different from how the items are worded on the checklist (to determine how the SPs respond when an item is phrased in a manner requiring them to interpret its meaning).
- Work in questions that require simple one-word answers (closed-ended questions) with those that require the SPs to give a more detailed explanation (open-ended questions) in order to give them practice in volunteering only appropriate checklist information.
- Portray students with more or less sensitivity to the patient's circumstances (to give the SPs practice in expressing their reactions within a range of appropriate emotional responses).
- Eliminate from each practice encounter various questions and physical exam maneuvers found on the checklist (to ascertain how accurate the SPs are when recording what happened).
- Do physical exam maneuvers correctly and incorrectly; perform them in a different order each time, add physical exam maneuvers that are not on the checklist, and so on.
- Share information in different styles and purposefully include and exclude certain information.
- Educate the patient about needed lifestyle changes with varying degrees of skill, from masterful to confusing (to give the SPs practice in writing comments from the patient's perspective about how successful the student's efforts were with the patient).

This mixing of techniques will prepare your SPs better than anything else for the variety of interactions they will inevitably experience with the students they encounter during the clinical examination.

In closing, Table 2.1 summarizes the skill sets needed by the SP coach and the standardized patients as discussed in this chapter.

Table 2.1   Summary of Requisite Skills for the Coach and the SPs

Skill Areas	SP Coach's Skills	SPs' Skills
History Taking (HX)	Take a medical history. Interview a patient.	Memorize the facts of the case. Determine when and how much information to deliver during an exam without inappropriately volunteering information.
Physical Exam (PE)	Reproduce simulated PE findings. Coach the SPs into authentically reproducing the PE simulations. Perform all the required PE maneuvers on the checklist correctly and incorrectly. Perform other maneuvers that students are likely to perform.	Accurately and realistically simulate physical findings. Accurately determine whether the student performed the PE maneuvers correctly.
Patient-Physician Interaction/ Communication Skills (PPI)	Perform a range of communication skills without going to unrealistic extremes.	Accurately assess the students' communications skills on the PPI scale.
Information Sharing/Patient Education (IS)	Perform a range of different styles in delivering a variety of information to the patient.	Respond and negotiate with the medical students within the agreed upon parameters.
Performance	Coach the emotional/ psychological aspects of the SPs' performances. Simulate a wide range of medical students with the SPs.	Perform the emotional/ psychological aspects of the patient in a realistic manner. Take direction from the SP coach. Observe student behaviors while performing each encounter and accurately recall and record student behaviors on the checklists.
Feedback	Provide feedback to the SPs on their performances.	Give effective feedback to each medical student.

CHAPTER SUMMARY

This chapter has presented specific suggestions for helping the SP coach (who does not have a background in clinical medicine) to acquire enough ability in the four basic sets of clinical skills so that the coach has the foundation necessary to effectively train his or her standardized patients. These basic skill sets include:

- history taking.
- physical examination.
- patient–physician interaction or communication skills.
- information sharing or patient education skills.

These four basic clinical skill sets have been delineated in this chapter with the intent that an aspiring SP coach will develop enough expertise in these areas to assist the SPs in learning to make sound performance choices when working with a variety of students. In particular, this chapter provides specific directions and resources for acquiring many of the doctoring skills the medical students are learning. Knowing these skills is particularly important because the coach must model them during practice encounters by playing the role of the medical student with the SPs. The chapter also offers detailed techniques whereby the coach can implement these skills with the standardized patients.

LOOKING AHEAD

The next two chapters (Chapter 3—Acting: Understanding How the SPs Portray the Patient and Chapter 4—Directing: Coaching to Deepen the SPs Performances) illustrate how you can incorporate many of the techniques from the dramatic arts into your repertoire of skills as an SP coach. In doing so, you can help your SPs create patient portrayals that are so real that, for the most part, the medical students will forget they are interacting with SPs—or that they are performing with actors in a clinical examination where there are cameras and where they are being graded. As a result of such authenticity, the students will be more likely to work with the SPs in the same way that they work with the real patients they encounter in the clinics and hospitals where they are doing their training. The resulting authenticity in the *students'* own clinical performances is one of the key reasons we need to work so diligently to assist our SPs in attaining such impeccable performances and portrayals.

CHAPTER THREE

Acting: Understanding How the SPs Portray the Patient

Coaching standardized patients on the emotional and psychological aspects of a patient case (including the production of believable simulated physical findings) requires a different set of skills from the clinical skills described in the previous chapter. This is why it is so useful for us to understand something about the actor's process. Although it is certainly not necessary to be an actor or to have formally studied acting in order to effectively train SPs, it is advantageous—and will bring a deeper understanding to the work we are doing—if coaches have had the direct experience of performing a few standardized patient cases themselves. Such firsthand experience provides a clear, immediate understanding of all aspects of preparing for a performance, as well as insight into what the SPs face in bringing a patient to life.

This chapter presents some of the tools of the acting profession with the intent of providing insight into the actor's process and guides you through several exercises to assist you in understanding how the emotional and psychological elements of a patient case can be evoked. In the latter part of the chapter, I have used the actor's process as a model for how we might think about our work with SPs, especially during the preparation phase leading to performance. Throughout, I have included insights from well-known actors and directors.

GETTING INTO THE PATIENT'S PSYCHE

Essentially this chapter is about how actors do what they do—about how SPs take on the qualities of the patient they are portraying. Acting is about more than learning lines and character development. It is about getting into patients' psyches—their emotional and psychological make-up—in order for the SP to give rise to an entirely believable portrayal of the patient during each encounter of a clinical exam.

What It Is Like to Be a Patient

All patients—real or standardized—in certain key aspects of their relationship to their doctor need to get what they want through someone else. That is part of the uneasiness of being a patient. The patient has to depend on the doctor who may or may not understand his concerns and what he is going through. This is at the core of every patient case your SPs will play, every patient case you, as a coach, will develop. Patients do not have many options, nor do they have much control in the clinical setting. They are often anxious or angry, frightened or frustrated, cajoling or manipulative, all of which determines how they act toward the doctor. For instance, if the patient is frustrated because of the way he was treated on previous visits to the doctor's office, he might show his frustration by demanding things of the doctor he otherwise would not. Therefore, the SP's intention in playing a patient will not only be colored by the patient's personality but also by the very nature of the patient's dependence on the doctor for whatever it is he wants or needs.

Something else to think about is that the patient's complexity as a human being generally shows itself through the multiplicity of styles of interactions the SPs have with various medical students. Therefore, the specifics of how the SP should respond to every eventuality cannot be pinned down on paper (like the written dialogue and directions in a play or film script). However, this does not mean that there cannot be limits. For example, you can tell the SP that no matter what happens in an encounter, he is not allowed to display anger or leave the room. So there can be parameters on the SP's actions that still allow him to respond to what is alive in the moment-to-moment shifts of every clinical encounter.

The Patient Case: The Foundation of SP Performance

Every case has emotional and psychological components, whether or not they are explicitly described in the training materials. This concept is sometimes overlooked in the development of SP cases, yet these components are the foundation on which the final performance depends. In our work, we must have a sense of these facets of the patient in order to accurately select persons who are appropriate to portray the case. If we are hiring non-actors, we need to know the natural qualities to look for, that is, the qualities in the potential SP that mirror the patient's characteristics. Likewise, these very components of the case are the heart of what the SP will use to create the portrayal of the patient—and are therefore critical to the case, even if the case authors have not described them in the case materials. I say this emphatically because our job as coaches is to train our SPs to take on the characteristics of real people. All patients, no matter what their medical problem, have both emotional and psychological elements that are integral to their personalities. These elements are important whether they are intended to be immediately apparent in the proposed simulated clinical encounter or not.

Portraying Real Patients

All simulated patient cases should be based on real patients. This principle is basic to the development of a strong, authentic case. The reasoning behind this principle is to keep case development focused on actual patient experiences rather than on contrived, abstract situations. In addition, if possible, the patient on whom the case is being developed should be known to one or another of the case authors, who are usually faculty physicians. This allows the author to refer to actual situations that occurred with the patient whenever questions arise about the physical, emotional, and psychological make-up of the patient.

Emotional and psychological qualities are core elements of being human and are thus the components that give each patient his or her unique and, at the same time, universal characteristics. Therefore, if we and our SPs train without looking for, and without a common understanding of, these underpinnings of the patient's personality, we run the risk of ending up with nonstandardized performances that come out of fabrications about the patient that are not only unspoken but perhaps not even reflected on.

FAMILIARIZING OURSELVES WITH THE ACTOR'S TOOLS

To acquire an understanding of the fundamental skills that actors use, the obvious place to look is to the acting profession itself and to well-known actors and directors. As coaches, we can then apply this knowledge to our training of SPs, as well as to our own portrayals when we are playing the role of a medical student in the SPs' training sessions.

The tools I discuss here are the very ones that have been discovered and used again and again by actors and directors all over the world. They are the techniques that naturally emerge when we search for them because they come out of our basic make-up as human beings. In our day-to-day lives, most of us are not aware of our deepest motivations or of the feelings and behaviors that are triggered by these influences—because for most daily activities we need not be consciously aware of these things. But to give a truly realistic performance, our SPs must comprehend what is going on in the patient's psychology. At the very least, the SPs need to understand the following elements (which should be explicitly defined in the training materials):

- *needs*—what the expressed and unexpressed needs of the patient are.
- *expectations*—what the patient wants or anticipates getting out of the clinical visit.
- *fears*—if relevant to the case, what the patient is anxious or worried about.

Equally important for the SPs is to understand their own psychology, that is, what is going on inside themselves at the time of their portrayal. The importance of this understanding stems from their need to reproduce certain states of being (with which they are internally familiar) when they are called for in their work. This ability—to tap into and capture in themselves the specific manifestations of the human experience called for in the patient they are portraying—is the measure of their skill and the nature of the actor's craft.

The core of acting is a study in human motivation. For the SPs it is a study of the patient's motivation—and their own. In fact, this is the baseline for anyone who wants to portray someone else. There are many ways to achieve this end. However, as in the field of acting, there is much debate in the field of standardized patient training about which method works best in order to act or to direct actors to portray a patient or to coach SPs. There are as many people using other methods as there are those who follow "The Method."[1] But, it seems that the emphasis is in the wrong place. For our purposes, this debate does not really matter. What does matter is the final effect of whatever method we choose. Most people looking at a painting do not care whether the painter used a knife, dripped the paint on the canvas, or used a brush. What matters is the effect of the painting on the viewer. What matters for us is the effect of the SP's portrayal on the medical student. The particular means the SP and the coach use to achieve this end is less important, which is not to say

---

[1] The Method is the most well-known epithet in the field of acting. Its most famous proponent was Marlon Brando. The Method was first established by Stanislavsky to replace the dated histrionic style of acting that was common at the turn of the 20th century with a more naturalistic kind of acting whereby the actor uses his own inner experiences to portray a character.

that one should disregard the many who have gone before and opened the way for us to learn, experiment, and acquire techniques of our own.

For this reason, at the end of this book I have provided a list of additional readings on acting, which can give you a more in-depth background on this subject. These readings collectively represent a variety of methods that have been developed out of Russian-born actor/director Constantin Stanislavsky's original work and, at the same time, give a sense of the multiplicity of skills that can be used to support a performance. Listed, as well, in the additional readings are texts on directing for stage, film, and television, which can be adapted for work with SPs. You might also find it interesting and informative to watch the weekly television program *Inside the Actors Studio* in which famous actors are interviewed about their craft, and relevant clips are shown from their films—amid an enthusiastic audience of acting and directing students.

THE INTERCONNECTEDNESS OF ACTING, DIRECTING, AND SP COACHING

Living truthfully under imaginary circumstances . . . .
—Sanford Meisner (Meisner & Longwell, 1987, p. 15)

In this epigraph, Meisner, one of the seminal figures in the development and teaching of contemporary acting techniques, captures succinctly what all actors are striving for. The notion of living truthfully under imaginary circumstances works equally well as a guidepost for us and our SPs. We, too, are striving to help our SPs live genuinely in the moment (not falsely by preconceived ideas) under the imaginary circumstances of a simulated clinical encounter so that their performances have the spontaneous ring of truth to them.

It is easy to detect a contrived performance, but the mystery is just what exactly goes into making up an authentic SP portrayal from the SP's, as well as the coach's, point of view. And so, we will explore how and what actors and directors do to bring a character to life so that we can learn from them and the dramatic arts—in other words, from the profession that is closest to what we do as coaches. It is my hope that this understanding of acting will help you shape your SPs' portrayals into the kind of performances you are looking for.

As I was thinking about our work with standardized patients, the image came to mind of a dolmen—those prehistoric megaliths of two standing stones supporting a capstone that is always exquisitely balanced across them. So, too, I envision that what we do as SP coaches rests on the professional work already crafted by actors and directors. I see

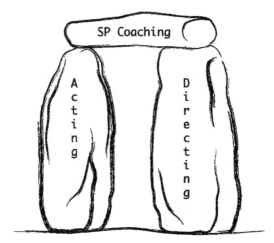

Figure 3.1 The Stones of the Dolmen.

the means by which directors tend and actors accomplish the goal of living truthfully in their performances as the supporting stones—and the manner in which we intuitively coach our SPs, using knowledge from both of these fields as the bridge stone resting on the two foundation stones. This structure creates a portal—a way through and into the unexplored, the unfolding of the process that we experience every time SPs and their coaches come together to create something new. Figure 3.1 represents this interrelationship.

SPs as Actors, Coaches as Directors

From the early 1960s, when standardized patients were first used in medical education, to now, our work with SPs has depended on the dramatic arts. In essence, we are all actors whether we are aware of it or not—or whether we have formal training in acting or not.

Acting is defined simply as "to play the part of" (*The American Heritage College Dictionary*, 1997). However, Meisner's epigraph refines the definition of what the art of acting has meant since the early part of the 20th century when Stanislavsky developed a system of acting based on the insights he discovered while working with his fellow actors at the Moscow Art Theatre in Russia. With his encouragement of a more natural, realistic style of acting, Stanislavsky became the first to define the actor's art as we know it today. During his lifetime, his influence went well beyond Russia into Europe and America. Then with the growth of global culture at the end of the 20th century, his principles continued to find their way around the world inspiring many others to seek their own particular ways to help actors realistically express the inner lives of the characters they are playing. The universal acting qualities that Stanislavsky defined still inspire and shape the craft wherever actors and audiences come together around the world—in film, in television, or on the stage. And now we, too, are included in this alliance.

Whether we are working with standardized patients who are trained actors or not, we are all tending the actor's craft. As we coach our standardized patients and support them in their efforts to bring alive their own creativity in the service of the patient they are portraying, our work is comparable to that of all other actors and directors. Our job as their coach is to support the SPs in using their own instruments—their own bodies, their own being, their own talents and imagination to create performances that are indistinguishable from the look and feel of a real patient. However, before we explore the specifics of the art of acting as related to coaching SP performances, it is important to look at other basic considerations.

Blending Standardization With the Creative Process

How we interpret the meaning of standardization in our work is crucial. This understanding is just as important for how we adjust the acting part of the SP's performance as it is for how we calibrate the SP's performance of simulated physical findings, which usually have some psychological element or emotion attached to them. (Think about the psychological adjustment needed because of the physical deficits caused by a stroke or the emotional component of pain.) When talking about the creativity of preparing to play a role, Stanislavsky (1958/1999) used the analogy of planting a seed that must sprout and flower by first taking root in the soul of the actor, this being the moment that the creative process begins (p. 183). Each time we work with an SP case, something new and alive will arise if we allow the SPs to participate in the process of making the patient case their own, of allowing that seed to grow in the soil of their own being. This is a good thing—even though we are working toward standardization—because the truth is, no performance is ever like any other performance, even when the actors have to speak the same memorized lines in a play, because it is not solely the words that make the performance. It is even less so in the improvised situation we are training our SPs to work in.

How can standardized patients be allowed to bring something fresh to the case each time it is trained—or, for that matter, each time it is performed? Using the actor's craft to evoke feelings from the core of her being, the SP must then stay constantly in touch with what is going on inside herself, as well as with what is going on outside herself during the interaction, in order to allow those elements that relate to the case to emerge as words or actions. This is what lies at the heart of "living truthfully under imaginary circumstances." This is what keeps a case, a performance, alive. This is true for every artist whether musician, writer, dancer, painter, or actor. The moment of performance must have that sense of spontaneity that is part of every living being who has a nervous system. We are constantly sensing and feeling things in slightly different ways, from moment to moment. Not to honor the ability (the SP's natural gift), the craft, the discipline that can put the SP in touch with that spontaneity is to settle for only getting by, when we can encourage the so-much-more of what I have just described.

So, in this creative context, what does it mean when we talk about standardization of a case? Standardization has to do with the SPs providing the same challenge for each examinee taking the clinical exam. However, within this standardization guideline, there can be variation of expression in the patient portrayal. For instance, if the SP case requires the medical student to deal with the emotional aftermath of telling the patient she has breast cancer, then there must be leeway in the manner in which the patient expresses the emotion she is feeling on hearing the bad news. The SPs' performances will be much more real if the behavior expressed comes from the natural unfolding of the emotion in the context of what is happening in the encounter—so long as the challenge remains the same for every medical student who interacts with the SP. Our job as coaches is to give feedback to the SPs, during training and throughout the clinical skills examination, about how their performances are coming across and whether or not what they are doing remains true to the character of the patient under the specific circumstances they are facing with the person interacting with them. These are the elements that define a performance; some are fluid, whereas others are constant. SPs can be coached into standardized performances with this kind of sensitivity, which simultaneously ensures that each student will face a patient who embodies the same degree of difficulty.

Providing the same challenge in the simulated clinical encounter is often confused with the notion that standardization has something to do with requiring each SP to manifest the same, fixed external behaviors so that their performances look exactly alike to the student. This is a misconception that almost guarantees a lifeless performance, lacking the spark of truth we are aiming for. Not only this, but even more fundamental is the fact that a total standardization of performances is not possible— even if spontaneity is not a value—whether the performances of a specific case are given by a single individual SP or by multiple SPs, because of the following factors:

- Since the students' actions and reactions themselves are not standardized, the SP must respond to whatever the medical student spontaneously does during the clinical encounter.
- No matter how successful we are at selecting SPs who have similar physical characteristics to play the same case, their personalities will inevitably be different, and it is out of their individuality that the responses of the patient they are portraying must emerge. Where else can they go for the touchstone of emotional understanding but to themselves, their own observations, their own experiences?

Furthermore, the conviction that requiring the SPs to use specific predetermined behaviors can produce performances that are not only uniform but also come across as consistently believable has embedded in it a misconceived assumption: that an *idea* about how a person would behave under certain circumstances, imposed by an act of will, is synonymous with reliably realistic performances.

The truth is, we *can* have SP performances that are both realistic *and* standardized if we adhere to these principles:

- All SPs must understand the patient's character and motivations in the same way.
- The SPs must be able to tap into the place of feeling within themselves (out of which the patient's behavior can naturally materialize) by whatever means or techniques work for them.
- The SPs must have the courage to allow those actual responses/feelings to manifest appropriately based on what is going on in the clinical encounter.

At this point you might ask, "What if I don't work with people who can do this?" Or worse yet, "What if I don't know *how* to work with people who can do this?" In this chapter and the next (on directing), I address the concerns behind these questions, but first let me bring another important consideration out of the shadow and into the spotlight—the actor/non-actor issue.

Actor/Non-Actor Considerations

All things considered, training standardized patients to give good portrayals is a rather forgiving business. Why? Because most of us are rather good at telling stories. It is what we do all the time when we recount any experience to another person. It is what most patients want to do when they go to see the doctor. Many cases simply call for an SP who can learn the facts and tell the story while being himself. A seemingly simple requirement—until we find ourselves working with someone who has trouble playing himself when he has to *perform* as the patient.

There are two main reasons why this happens: either the SP—actor or non-actor—becomes too self-conscious to let go into her imagination and feelings, or she tries too hard and ends up "acting" an idea or a stereotype of the patient. (Note that this ineffective way of operating can be self-imposed just as easily as it can be imposed from the outside by the SP coach.) In either case, believability is usually sacrificed. The antidote to this situation lies in our expertise in choosing SPs by their ability, natural or acquired, to relate the experience of the patient "as if" it were a story about themselves. It also lies in the SP coach having enough grounding in acting and directing to be able to help the SPs shape their portrayals when that is what is called for.

Another important quality to look for in an SP is the ability to shift the focus from himself (self-consciousness is the root of performance anxiety) to the person with whom the SP is interacting. If the SP can tell the patient's story as if it were his own and focus more on the student and her reactions than on himself, we have someone we can work with.

Once again, what we are talking about here is how to "live truthfully under imaginary circumstances." In terms of authenticity of performance, the coach's job is to support the SPs' internal work so that their portrayals continue to be true to the character and circumstances of the patient. It is not about encouraging portrayals that are based on preperformance notions regarding how the patient is supposed to perform at certain points in the encounter, such as jiggling a leg to indicate discomfort when the student pursues a particular line of questioning that is supposed to make the patient uneasy (such as an alcohol, substance use, or sexual history). In fact, most SPs working out of this model will in all probability produce performances that appear false, overacted, or artificial—in other words, they end up "acting-with-a-capital-A." It is these kinds of performances that have alienated so many in our field from working with actors. But acting-with-a-capital-A can happen just as easily with non-actors as it can with unskilled actors. The whole issue is about a performance that rings true—a performance that is not too big or too forced or too on-the-surface. It is about a performance that is spontaneous—one that, like water, flows with and on the rising of relevant internal feelings that are appropriate to what is happening at any given moment in the encounter. An SP who does not have any formal training in acting can potentially do this as skillfully as one who does have a background in acting.

As a general rule, however, non-actors are best used for cases in which there are no emotional or psychological challenges, and the SPs can simply play themselves. The way most of us choose an SP for these kinds of situations is to pick a person whose basic personality fits the case description. We hire a naturally talkative person if the case requires that quality; we steer away from hiring a quiet, shy person for such a case. Remember also that other quality that we should be looking for—unselfconsciousness. Actually, more than that, we should be looking for someone who is not only at ease, but who blossoms when telling the patient's story in front of other people. And always, always we must remain alert and open to discovering the natural—the non-actor who has some innate ability to take on patient characteristics that are very unlike herself, that are outside her own personality.

The best way to discover these qualities is through auditioning, in which we have face-to-face interactions with our potential recruits, using the specific case materials in question. It is through this auditioning process that we get a taste of the performance qualities each recruit possesses, a feel for how it might be to give them direction, and what it will be like to work with each of them (see chapter 5, Casting: Finding the Right Standardized Patients, for more on auditioning).

No doubt you have already surmised that whenever possible, I prefer to work with persons who have both some natural talent and some training in acting. If the case I am training has strong emotional or deep psychological elements necessary for the portrayal, I will first look for a skilled actor because a case of this sort requires the SP not only to have the skill to create a credible performance from more demanding requirements but also to be able to consistently produce this performance time after time, student after student. It takes a certain kind of mastery to believably play an emotion again and again as if it were the first time the patient has experienced it. Although it is possible on occasion for a non-actor who has innate talent to achieve this quality of performance, it is much more difficult for the non-actor to *maintain* such a performance. Therefore, working with non-actors in these circumstances will require significantly more monitoring and coaching of the SPs in their work with the medical students than would be necessary with capable, trained actors. It is often possible to coach a non-actor into a single performance that works well, but likely during a clinical exam the coach will not have enough time to devote to someone who cannot internally re-create the situation on her own.

As one might imagine, to develop this kind of performance skill takes practice. Proficient actors come with techniques and expertise that have become second nature to them, all of which means we will not have to do the work the SP should be doing in order to get the kind of performance we are looking for.

However, coaches not familiar with working with SPs who have a background in acting usually feel some trepidation about the prospect of interacting with them. It is helpful to remind ourselves that we do not need to go so far as to take on the responsibility of teaching our SPs how to act. Our job is to be a *coach* of our SPs' performances. Therefore, we must learn about the various ways SPs may go about producing their portrayals so that we are able to offer appropriate suggestions (relevant to their style of working) that help them adjust their performances. Then along the way, as we learn about various acting techniques we might occasionally want to introduce one or another of them to an SP when it seems appropriate to do so. However, if the SP cannot produce the performance we are looking for, or cannot be consistent or take direction, we have a problem—and one that probably will not go away no matter how much time and effort we put into their training—or how much we learn about acting and directing.

Even if the case does not demand a high degree of acting expertise, a well-chosen actor will always be able, on his own, to find elements in the character of the patient that help him flesh out his portrayal. If you know the patient case well enough to have a sense of what you want to see in the SP's performances, if you are sincere in your efforts to communicate that vision, and if you have created a trusting relationship in which you can be honest when you do not know how to communicate something in their language, actors will help you learn how to give them what they need. Your working relationship with your actors then creates an opportunity for you to experiment and grow in your coaching skills. So if you can gather into your SP pool even a small cadre of capable actors and on your own acquire some basic knowledge about what it is that actors do, and what they need from us in training, the task of coaching your SPs' performances will be much easier and more rewarding.

THE ART OF ACTING: A MODEL FOR ENHANCING PATIENT PORTRAYALS

If we truly wish to enhance our SPs' portrayals, we need to understand how actors produce performances that look and feel spontaneously real—and how we as their coaches can help our SPs in this pursuit. In fact, the more we know about how actors work, the better we will be at coaching our SPs into the kind of performances we are looking for. To provide better support for our SPs, let's begin with learning something about acting, represented by one of the standing stones in the dolmen. By looking at how actors produce a believable performance, we can discern more keenly the relationship between the actor's craft and what our SPs can do to create realistic patient portrayals. We start by looking at two contemporary approaches often used by actors to create a role—the *outside-in* approach and the *inside-out* approach.

Within these two approaches there are many schools of thought, but Stanislavsky is the most significant modern figure whose work is the source of a number of present-day acting methods. What Stanislavsky was seeking when he began systematically observing the most accomplished actors of his day—talking with them about how they prepared for a role, trying those things out for himself, inventing others—was to formulate his experiences into a system that could be of practical use to others. Stanislavsky's system is sometimes associated exclusively with the inside-out approach, but in fact he incorporated both points of view. The system he devised did not come out of an abstract theory, but directly from the experience of actors, which is no doubt why it is still valuable today. In what follows, you will find a sampling of Stanislavsky's methods, along with examples of other techniques that are relevant to these two approaches and to our work with SPs. The approach an actor identifies with is the one that is most comfortable for her based on her own personality type, but no matter which approach an actor feels most drawn to, the techniques she uses in her process of creating a performance need to bring her to conscious or unconscious internal images that evoke the feeling she is seeking to portray.

Working From the Outside-In: Using Observed Behaviors to Develop Character

The outside-in approach refers to creating a performance by observation of self and others to pick up external manifestations—the details, the particularities of behavior that can be used in defining character. It is considered by many to be predominantly a system based on technical expertise, that is, on the use of body, movement, gesture, and voice.

The outside-in approach can be particularly helpful if the actor is playing a character who is quite different from himself. SPs might find this process useful whenever they are required to play a patient whose life and experiences are unlike anything the SP has experienced in his own life—say a patient who has a mental disorder or an adolescent who is living on the street and having to resort to prostitution to survive. As the foundation for creating their portrayals with these kinds of cases, the SPs might want to do some research. They might read books or watch a video of a patient with the mental disorder the SP is going to portray—or perhaps visit a psychiatric ward where the SP might observe such a patient in interaction with others, to see how the mental disorder manifests in the patient's behavior. If an SP playing the street kid were to use this approach, he might go to a part of the city where someone living this lifestyle spends much of his time. He might hang out with such kids to get a sense of what makes them tick. In this way, he might pick up some unique qualities that he would want to try on himself as he works out his patient portrayal.

Classically trained British actors are prime examples of performers who work from this approach. When asked how he shaped a performance, Lawrence Olivier talked about the need to "collect a lot of details, a lot of characteristics, and find a creature swimming about somewhere in the middle of them" (Cottrell, 1975, p. 389). Olivier further elaborated,

> The actor persuades himself first, and through himself, the audience. In order to achieve that...you've got...to scavenge the tiniest little bit of circumstance; observe it; find it, use it some time or other.... I've got a memory for little details. I've had things in the back of my mind for as long as eighteen years before I've used them...In the years that follow, you wonder what it was that made them do it, and ultimately, you find in that the illuminating key to a whole bit of characterization. (Cottrell, p. 388)

In the last part of Olivier's explanation is the hint of his desire to also understand what was going on internally with the person who produced those bits of behavior: "...you wonder what it was that made them do it, and ultimately, you find in that the illuminating key...." From his wondering about the behavioral details he had observed came the internal perception that Olivier used to re-create the character. Here is another way Olivier expressed the melding of the external circumstances he observed with the internal work he did in his search for the character he was to play: "Well, I ask myself, 'Who do I know like that?' It might be me, but it might be a dozen other people as well" (Cottrell, p. 390).

"Who do I know like that?" Like what? Like who the person is whose external behaviors tell us something about them or what they are experiencing. This approach to characterization begins with the cognitive, moves to objective reality (those behavioral bits of circumstance), all of which end up stimulating the imagination inside the actor. The internal and the external are like the two sides of a coin, each side integral to the whole.

Practically speaking, how do the external and the internal work in concert with each other? The exercises that follow are intended to give an appreciation of how each aspect combines with the other in the process of creating a complete performance. By getting a taste of what actors do and experience, directors can better interact with them when their performances do not live up to their vision of the character. This same kind of experiential understanding can help us define our own performance expectations, our own role when working with our SPs.

I encourage you not only to read what follows, but also to try these exercises so that you can experience the effect they can have on you. I guarantee that your experience will be different from what you expect— and what happens may even amaze you.

An Outside-In Exercise to Evoke Emotional States

For the next day or so, consciously look at people's behaviors. A good place to do this is in a public setting, such as a gym or a coffee shop where you can be anonymous. Do this by yourself so that you can concentrate on the exercise. Keep a notebook handy to jot down details. Scan the room until something about someone stops you—in other words, until something about someone intrigues you. Note what it is about the person that arouses your interest. Literally write down the details that are attracting your attention. Stay with the objective, observable behaviors of the person. You may find that the person has mannerisms that are endearing or annoying, that she is wearing clothes you like or dislike or find unique and interesting, and so on. At this point, try not to get caught up in the *effect* that these observations are having on you. Simply register these interpretations in the back of your mind and stay focused on the tangible, external manifestations. For the moment, what matters is what you are objectively discerning in her look, in her behavior, and in the way she carries herself, the way she walks, the way she is sitting. If you are close enough to hear what the person is saying, listen to the tone in her voice, listen to her inflections, and the rhythm of her speech. Keep writing down all of this so that you can repeat these behaviors later on. Don't give up until something surprises you, until something emerges out of the pieces you are collecting that you were not aware of at first.

Once you have written down a number of bits and pieces about the person's behavior, shift your attention to what is going on inside yourself. You might find it easier "to go inside" if you close your eyes. Now is the time to focus on the interpretations you put on hold and on any stories about the person that her behavior spawned in your imagination. Go further yet, stay curious, and ask yourself what these bits are telling you about the person's possible motivations, about what she might want or need from the other people she is interacting with. In other words, "wonder what it was that made them do it."

Now, shift gears and ponder the circumstances that might be defining the person's actions, meaning anything in the environment that might be influencing her behavior. It could be the physical setting, the fact that the person has her arm in a sling, or that he is sitting between two women who are talking over him, or that she has another appointment (she has looked at her watch twice since you've been observing her). If there's no way to know what some of the circumstances are, fantasize what they might be.

This is the process that occurs whenever we make up stories about people. This is the process we and our SPs should be going through when we are initially analyzing the training materials for a patient case. These circumstances are often the most crucial influences on behavior. This layering of understanding coming out of our curiosity about the person and her circumstances is some of the most important material actors work with to create a portrayal—no matter which approach (outside-in or inside-out) they have an affinity for.

All right, you have collected your data, you have noted your own stories and interpretations about the person and you have pondered his circumstances. It's time to pick out several bits of behavior that seem to define the person in that setting. Make a separate list of them and reflect on them as you write them down. Why, in your mind, are these bits of behavior, and not others, the defining characteristics of the person?

Now comes the fun part, the part that will reveal the fruits of all your work. Once you feel satisfied with your list, it's time to practice using what you have observed. Away from the setting where you have collected your data, try out one or two of the behaviors as you talk to yourself in the mirror. Really, try it—no one's watching but you! You don't have to be a Meryl Streep or a Robert de Niro to do this. Then find an opportunity to try a combination of these behaviors in a monologue with yourself (or a dialogue with an imaginary companion) in the privacy of your home—or when you're stuck in traffic. See what happens by taking on the external behaviors of the person you have observed. What you will probably discover is that in using these external behaviors, something will stir inside you, something different from what you experienced in watching the person, something different from what you *thought* was going on inside that person. Keep going, keep dialoguing, and allow whatever is happening to grow and take on a life of its own. See what images emerge. Be aware of what's happening in your body. Are there any new sensations, any tensions you hadn't noticed before—anything from your facial expressions to the gripping of the toes in your shoes?

The truth this exercise brings out is that there is really no separate inside and outside reality. The notion of splitting reality into two parts is simply an abstract concept. It's not how we *experience* reality. How we feel inside is directly related to how we perceive what is happening on the outside, and how we experience the external world directly influences how we are feeling internally.

At this point, it is important to distinguish the difference between the outside-in approach just illustrated and the cookbook approach that we sometimes see in standardized patient work. The systematized wring-your-hands-to-show-anxiety approach is quite different from using the outside-in technique to access a patient's true feelings (which I hope you have gotten a little feel for here). Such preconceived, generic ideas about how to express an emotional state come from stereotypes that, in the name of standardization, become fixed behaviors that can kill the aliveness of the performance. By contrast, the outside-in approach is a different means of "living truthfully under imaginary circumstances," another way to access the emotion the SP is seeking in her portrayal.

True standardization in using the outside-in approach is produced out of an understanding of the patient's emotional truth that each SP discovers inside herself by working with external behaviors she has actually observed in herself or someone else—or, better yet, behavior she has observed in a real patient. Experimenting with these observed behaviors opens up a process of discovery. The SP finds the emotional truth of the patient through images that arise out of working with these bits of relevant external behavior that originally expressed an internal state of being.

Physical Control of the Body and Voice

Not only must an SP be able to produce the physical findings called for by the part she is playing during the physical examination (and perhaps throughout the encounter), but her body must also be able to respond to the appropriate emotional impulses that arise in her as she plays the patient and produces those physical findings. This is what Stanislavsky (1999) was referring to when he talked about "the perfecting of a physical apparatus"—the body—which then would be at the service of the actor no matter what his role demanded of him physically. He also did not want the body to hinder the imagination by not being able to perform whatever was called for or needed to emerge, spontaneously (p. 189).

The same is true of the voice. All performers (in fact, all of us) know the power of the tone of voice to convey the content of words—or to deny the content of the words when we are trying to camouflage the feeling behind the words. Stanislavsky's intent was to move the actor away from a predetermined manner of delivery, away from one that was influenced by self-consciousness. This, of course, was consonant with the whole of his system. He was influenced by singers and musicians of all kinds in his approach to developing the voice so that it became, along with the physical body, an instrument of the imagination.

Physical control of the body and the voice is as critically important for SPs as it is for other performers. Think of how often SPs are required to simulate intricate external, physical findings at the same time that they must indicate internal conditions and concerns of the patient by the tone of their voice and the subtleties of their nonverbal behavior.

In the next section, we are going to look at another way of working from the "outside"—another way of using physical actions of the body and voice—in the service of getting in touch with internal feelings.

Using the Physical Correlates of Emotional States to Evoke Feelings

Anyone can bring into existence certain emotional states by reproducing, at will, the physical effects of a particular emotion. Here is the principle at work: Emotional states have physical correlates in the body, that is, the body responds physiologically in certain ways to particular feeling states that can be sensed in different ways. Each feeling state produces patterns of sensations in the body. For example, when we are anxious, our respiration can change with our breathing becoming shallower, faster, irregular; there can be a buzz of energy in the abdomen or the chest; the extremities can tingle or shake; the heart beats faster; the mouth gets dry; the muscles of the neck and throat constrict. And there are other even subtler physical changes that can be detected as one becomes more and more sensitive to particular emotional effects on the body. Most of the time we are unaware of these physical changes because the emotion either consumes us to the point that we get caught up in it as it intensifies, or because we try to make it go away by an automatic, learned reaction to stifle whatever it is we are feeling. We do this by either attempting to think or rationalize our way out of the feeling, or by doing something to distract ourselves from the unpleasantness of the feeling, such as changing the subject in a conversation, eating, smoking, having a drink, or watching television.

I have been focusing on unpleasant feelings, primarily because they are the emotions that patients are usually dealing with. Therefore, these are the feeling states our SPs need to be able to reproduce. Patients rarely go to a doctor because they are feeling well or are elated. But, if called for in a patient portrayal, positive energetic states can be elicited in exactly the same manner as I am about to describe.

There are many ways to coax a feeling into being. For the moment, let's look at the interconnectedness of the body, the emotions, and the mind. Some of the sensations related to emotions can be consciously controlled; others cannot. For instance, we can control the rate, depth, and regularity of our breathing, and the tension and relaxation of many of our muscles; we cannot directly will into being the sensation of tingling or a dry mouth. But in the process of manipulating some of the sensations, others will automatically emerge. For example, if we change our breathing, it can affect our heart rate. The reason for this is that there is a reciprocity among physical sensations, that is to say, physical sensations are interactive with each other. There is also a mutuality between physical sensations and internal feeling states. It goes both ways: Feelings create sensations in the body; physical sensations trigger other sensations and create feelings.

Knowing this, we can persuade genuine feelings to arise by playing with the sensations we have control over. As we change our breathing and tense our shoulders and neck, we will start to feel different. Because of this, it is important to be aware that while experiencing the changes in feeling states, one must be able to remain somewhat detached from those states. In other words, anyone using these techniques needs to be able to feel the physical sensations as well as the emotional feelings that arise and, at the same time, witness what is happening as if she were a scientist observing the effects of an experiment. Because consciously inducing feelings are not something we usually do in our everyday life, if we want to use these techniques with our non-actors, we must have a relationship of deep trust with them—even more than we do with our actor-SPs who likely have already worked with techniques similar to these in their training. Trust in us, as coaches, is essential for the SPs to be able to allow us to guide them through the process of consciously sensing and eliciting energies in the body that call up emotional states. Therefore, if you are not already familiar with these techniques and plan to use any of them with your SPs, I strongly encourage you to try the following exercises first so that you are acquainted with the territory.

Let's look at two common emotions that patients often bring into the clinical setting: anxiety and anger. (You might find it easier to stay focused during these exercises if you voice-record the instructions, then play them back when you are ready to actually try the exercises.)

Exercise to Induce Feelings of Anxiety

First, find a place to sit where you can be comfortable and still have freedom of movement. Close your eyes. Then when you are ready, start to change your breathing by inhaling and exhaling in a shallower, more rapid manner. After doing this for a minute or so, make the in-breath staccato and irregular. Repeat this a dozen or more times, keeping your eyes closed. Once you sense a rhythm, add irregularity to the out-breath as well. Play with these elements of your breathing just to see what happens—making the in-breath and the out-breath unbalanced in length and irregularity. (If at any time you feel uncomfortable with the exercise, simply open your eyes and go back to breathing normally. Return to the exercise when you feel you can.)

While keeping this breathing pattern going, round your shoulders and raise them toward your ears at the same time you are tensing the back of your neck and pushing down against your raised shoulders. Squeeze your eyes closed and exaggerate everything. You might now find tension in parts of your body you were not trying to manipulate—perhaps in your upper abdomen or your arms. You might also find yourself spontaneously bending over slightly or making sounds. As you do this, notice how you are feeling inside. You might actually feel more than anxiety; you might feel on the edge of fear. This might trigger a memory, some thoughts or images. Good. This is exactly what you want to have happen, so long as you are experiencing this in an impersonal way. You do not want to get caught up in the feelings to the point that you lose your ability to witness what is happening.

When you are ready, gradually release the tensions in your body one by one and allow your breathing to return to normal. Stay focused internally and note the sensations you are feeling. You might now be experiencing tingling in your chest or extremities or a buzzing sensation in your abdomen. Breathe normally for a minute or so. Continue to consciously relax any tension you sense in your body. When you feel ready, you can open your eyes.

In doing this preparatory exercise, you have come in contact with the full circle of how anxiety expresses itself through body sensations and in images and thoughts that surface in the mind. When we study the inside-out approach, we will explore how images and thoughts can be used as the primary sources to tap into physical sensations and feeling states. But for the moment, suffice it to say, when used effectively, any of these interactive elements can trigger the desired emotion. Before we look at the internal techniques, let's go through one more practical, physical example. The next exercise can be used to bring yourself to an understanding of how to get in touch with specific sensations and the feeling of anger.

Exercise to Induce Feelings of Anger

When looking at the physical effects of anger, what one notices most is that there is tension in the body. There are images and impulses to strike out at or to do harm to the person or thing that is creating the feeling of anger. One way to elicit this feeling of anger is to start out in a standing position with your eyes open. Then make a fist with your dominant hand and hit the open palm of the opposite hand again and again in a rhythmic fashion. Hit with intensity, but not to the point where you are hurting yourself. Tense up, glare at the wall, or imagine a person you are actually angry at, and allow your face to contort into a grimace. Clamp your jaws together. Squeeze your eyes closed and let sounds, grunts/growls come out of the physical feelings each time your fist hits its target. Open your eyes and start saying anything that comes into your mind that you might say to someone who's made you angry, for instance, "Don't you ever, ever, EVER do that again." Say this over a number of times, glowering at the wall or the person you're imagining, making it more and more intense (but don't scream—this is anger, not rage) until the change in internal feeling is obvious. Notice the tension in your voice and the grimace that's holding back the impulse to lose control. Then when you feel ready, speak as if the patient were answering questions the doctor would be asking.

Later, if you are working privately on a case with an SP, encourage him to keep hitting the palm of his hand. Let him grunt and growl as he responds to your statements and questions. Encourage the SP to let the feeling grow, but at the same time, let him know he is not to get to the point where he is hurting himself or anyone else. When you have gone through a bit of the encounter, coach the SP to stop the forced external activities and ask him to continue by holding and containing all the feelings that have arisen. Continue with the encounter. There should be an intensity that is palpable, but not over the top. If it is still too big for the needs of the encounter, coach him by telling him something like, "I want you to be angry, but I don't want you to frighten me." Keep working with him until you both sense he is performing where the patient needs to be.

To summarize, the intention of these exercises is to produce images and induce feelings by working with body sensations. "All well and good," you might be thinking, "but how is this supposed to work in the context of an SP encounter with a student?" Keep in mind that the process just described is only one of a number of means that can be used to produce desired internal feelings prior to performance. It is meant as a vehicle to put a person immediately in touch with underlying feelings that are similar to the patient's—so that the SPs are not performing the case out of stereotypes they might have. These are practice exercises. They are not meant to be used in the *midst* of a performance. They are meant as a means of helping the SP access specific feelings before the start of an encounter. If you are working with actors, they may already be using similar techniques on their own to prepare for their performances.

Such techniques may or may not be appropriate for use during a training session. If the SP is able to produce the emotion required, you do not need to do anything. However, such techniques are often helpful to use with SPs who have potential, but who simply cannot find the emotion called for during rehearsal. If you work with them individually, outside the formal training session, by guiding them through these kinds of exercises and having them play the encounter with you as soon as the feeling has been tapped into, it can help some SPs get to the place where they can elicit the feeling on their own. Once the SP has gotten in touch with the feeling, she must let the technique go, shift her focus to the feeling that has arisen, contain it, and allow it to carry her through her performance as the patient. A tall order, but very possible even with some non-actors who have the natural instinct, the courage, and the trust to put themselves in your hands as you coach them into feeling the sensations and emotions that arise. If you decide to work in this way, I suggest that before using any of these techniques with your SPs you ask their permission and do the work in private, especially with your non-actors.

Perhaps, you are wondering why it is important to exaggerate the sensations and feelings when doing these exercises. Why not just have the SP hit the emotional level needed and leave it at that? Remember, we are using this technique to help SPs who, left to their own devices, cannot access the feelings we are trying to help them get in touch with. What we are striving to achieve is to guide them in finding their own natural, instinctual way of expressing the particular emotion that is called for. Exaggeration helps the SPs become aware of what is going on physically, both externally and internally. Once that awareness is palpable, many SPs can then shift to working with subtler levels of the same energies.

Having said all of this, it is important to note one last thing. Some people will simply know how to realistically express the required emotion to your satisfaction without your having to do anything but describe what you are looking for. Of those who are having trouble, some will be able to work with you to produce performances that better fit what you want from them; others will be able to access and use the appropriate feelings by working with exercises such as the ones described in this chapter; and yet others might not be able to give you what you want no matter what you do. Therein lies the value of determining the prospective SP's ability to take direction during the auditioning phase of recruitment.

Working From the Inside-Out: Using the Imagination to Evoke Feelings

> Acting begins with a tiny inner movement so slight that it is almost completely invisible.... In early theatre rehearsals, the impulse may get no further than a flicker.... For this flicker to pass into the whole organism, a total relaxation must be there, either god-given or brought about by work.
> —Peter Brook (1968, p. 109)

In this section, we explore additional ways the actor can access that essential element, that almost imperceptible internal feeling—the "flicker" that director Peter Brook refers to. However, instead of working during the preparation phase with external manifestations that can put the actor in touch with an emotion (outside-in), this time we explore techniques designed to help the actor to tap into an emotion by starting from the inside, then working with the feeling until it manifests in a performance that is authentic and believable (inside-out). But before we move on, I would like to call your attention to Brook's honoring of the importance of relaxation, a state of being which is essential for the subtle energy of an emerging emotion to thrive. (I discuss this topic in more detail toward the end of the chapter.) In this quote, Brook also pays respect to natural ability as well as to skill hard won through training, just as we need to do in our work with standardized patients.

Let's start our inside-out exploration by looking at a few more of Stanislavsky's discoveries. Stanislavsky's system consists of identifying the practical aspects of acting that help the actor master the ability to get in touch with his inner creativity more often than if left to chance. The basis of this work involves helping the actor to get out of her own way when she is performing—to stop the destructive internal chatter ("How do I look?" "I'm no good." "What I'm doing sucks." "So-and-so's doing a better job than I am.")—and instead to use her awareness and her mind, during her preparation, to get in touch inside herself with the essence of the person she is to portray—to find that person in her own feelings, in her own being. Stanislavsky knew that without the development of skill and technique, an actor (or instinctive non-actor) might be able to give a single good performance on "inspiration," but that he could not consistently give the same quality of portrayal, performance after performance. This is, of course, as true of SPs working in the field of medicine as it is of actors who perform in other arenas.

In the following, as you read about the preparation and performance principles and techniques that I describe and relate to standardized patient work, remember that a complete understanding of each acting concept is dependent on familiarity with the other acting concepts. So, if you are new to these ideas about acting, try not to be discouraged if they do not make sense the first time you encounter them. Simply read through everything, get as much as you can, then go back, look at them again, and try them out on yourself with a case that requires an emotional response from the patient. Personally experiencing these acting principles—which come not only from Stanislavsky, but from a number of other actors and directors, and from standardized patients with whom I have worked over the years—will bring a different kind of understanding that is very helpful in building your confidence when you are faced with needing to find a way to assist an SP to give a performance that is closer to what you are looking for.

At this point, however, the task is simply for you to develop a core understanding of how actors prepare, using the inside-out approach, and what they do to produce and maintain a believable performance, without having to know the specific approach they are using to get there. The true value of this elemental understanding of how actors work will reveal itself as you try out various coaching techniques with your SPs later on. But for now we are still exploring what actors do so that you can call on that understanding when you need to help your SPs adjust their performances.

Preparation of the Patient Case

Although I discuss only a few specific aspects of an actor's preparation as applied to standardized patient work, preparation really includes everything from the first introduction of the patient case to the final rehearsal of the SPs before their performances in an actual exam. The first phase of SP preparation begins with an analysis of the training materials.

To paraphrase Stanislavsky, at this very early stage of preparation, as they work with the case materials, the coach and the SPs must form a partnership dedicated to discovering and bringing to light the case author's intentions "*and not replace them by their own inventions...*" (italics mine; Stanislavsky, 1999, p. 182).

Stanislavsky felt morally bound and was devoted to uncovering the true meaning of the play. He was committed, as he said, to the "exact and profound understanding of the spirit and thought of the playwright" (p. 182). For Stanislavsky, this work is the bedrock on which all else, done in the name of the play, rests. And so it must be for us and our SPs. This collective understanding of the case comes from more than simply reading through the training materials. An *analysis* of the materials is an integral part of the preparation both we and our SPs need to do in order to get ready for training and performance. What the coach and the SPs do in analyzing the training materials is very similar to what a director and actors do in analyzing a script. As coaches, we do some of this work alone before training begins. The SPs do some of it in conjunction with us at the first couple of training sessions, but they must do the rest on their own, between trainings. Moreover, if from our own analysis of the case, we keenly understand the nuances of the patient's character and the challenges built into the simulated clinical encounter, we will be able to guide the SPs' performances with ease—even when some of the SPs differ with us in their understanding of the case or their perceptions of the patient.

The Coach's Analysis of the Training Materials

Our analysis of the case takes place in two phases: First, by ourselves before training begins, followed by the analytical work we do with the SPs during the first session of training. The initial work we need to do is to analyze our "play" (the training materials) to understand (a) the purpose of the case, (b) the intentions of the authors, and (c) the built-in challenges to the medical students. From this careful consideration will emerge our vision of the clinical encounter and the standardization of the case. Our next responsibility is to (a) clearly communicate our vision to the SPs early in the training process and (b) listen to what the SPs themselves have gleaned from their initial reading of the training materials.

All discussions having to do with differences in case interpretation always need to take place on the foundation of the purpose of the case, the author's intentions, and the student challenges embedded in the case. Once "the spirit and thought" behind the case are collectively understood by the SPs, then, and only then, can they begin their own interior work. For the SP, it is about making personal the collective case understanding. She does this by melding her own insights about the patient, which she herself has mined from the materials, with the insights of her coach and her fellow SPs.

This requirement of working toward a collective interpretation of the patient to be portrayed is quite different from how actors normally work. Although actors typically shape their portrayals in keeping with their director's vision, just as the SPs do with their coach's, an actor's goal in other performance arenas would be to develop a portrayal that is distinctly her own and unlike anyone else's. It is important to keep this in mind when working with trained actors—particularly if you are sensing resistance in any of them—so that you can help them make the shift from acting based primarily on their individual, personal interpretation to working with other SPs and the coach in this unique collaborative way.

Similarly, if we do not do our homework as coaches, that is, allow the vision (the deep understanding of the case, the patient, and the student challenges) to take shape in us, the chances are strong that we will be all over the place when issues and differences of opinion arise among SPs during training. And it will be difficult, perhaps impossible, for us to be open to their creative interpretations, particularly when they materialize in performances that are different from what we imagined. The best way to honor our SPs' contributions is to be secure in our own vision of the encounter so that whenever we are surprised by their offerings, we have the confidence to step back and consider with openness whether what they have shown us will work with our analysis of the critical elements of the case.

One of the most important parts of our job as coaches is to be able to sense when an SP's portrayal of the case falls in line with our overall vision and the challenge of the case, *even though* we never thought about the portrayal manifesting in that particular way. When we are uncertain, we are often not open to other options—or we find ourselves sitting back and allowing an SP to continue performing the emotional aspects of a case in a manner that is simply not in keeping with how we envision the case even when our gut instincts are telling us that what the SP is doing is wrong. When we are not sure of ourselves, it is not easy to tell the SP that her performance is missing the mark, especially if we do not have a clue how to articulate and direct the SP into a performance that *is* what we want. The purpose of the material you find in this section is to bring you to a place where you not only feel capable of discerning when your SPs' performances are and are not—to paraphrase Stanislavsky again—"an exact and profound representation of the spirit and thought of the case author," but also to feel confident that you have the necessary skills to bring the SPs to that place when necessary.

Besides being essential to understanding the case with one mind (the substance and source of standardization), our individual and collective explorations of the written materials provide the first opportunity for us to connect with the SPs at a deeper level and to work with them in a creative and fluid environment while still keeping the training on track, interesting, and fun. Remember, no matter how detailed the training materials might be, there are always unanswered questions and new discoveries waiting to be uncovered in them.

The Coach's and SPs' Collective Analysis of the Training Materials

Although there are a number of ways to explore the training materials with the SPs, I suggest starting with these three questions:

- What do we understand about the patient's backstory?
- What are the SPs' assumptions about the patient (spoken or unspoken)?
- What are the patient's (the character's) expectations about the upcoming encounter with the doctor?

Whenever we think that we have verbally described our concept of the case well enough to the SPs, we frequently think that everyone has understood what we have said exactly as we meant it. More often than not, that is not the way it turns out—not necessarily because we are poor communicators, but because everyone perceives language from his or her own unique life experiences. If we do not explore the SPs' understanding of what we have said, we may be in for some big surprises when they start to perform the case. Consciously and sensitively evoking what the other person perceives is one of the core principles of communication—for us with our SPs, for the students with their patients, in fact for anyone communicating with anyone else. It is that generic.

What do we understand about the patient's backstory?   Specific kinds of questions that help us clarify who the patient is have to do with the patient's background, interests, family, job, and so on. This backstory is the touchstone for the SPs' work of bringing the patient to life and is another of the elements that contributes to case standardization. Encouraging the SPs to answer questions such as the following adds three-dimensionality to the patient as everyone collectively contributes to the shaping of the patient's backstory:

- What is the patient's typical day like? Has anything changed in his life as a result of his symptoms?
- Who does the patient live with? What kind of relationship does she have with each of these people? Who else belongs to her support system? What do *they* think of her symptoms?
- What did the patient do just before coming to the clinic? Does he have plans immediately after seeing the doctor? How will what the doctor says affect those plans? And so on....

These kinds of facts and details should be included in the training materials; however, if the backstory is missing or not sufficient, it falls to us to fill in the gaps. We can do this ourselves or we can solicit backstory from the SPs as we are working with them during the first training session. As you are already know, the only caveat is that the details must always support the case author's intentions.

What are the SPs' assumptions about the patient?   No matter how explicitly the backstory is laid out in the case materials, having an open discussion about the patient's background is essential. Simply asking each of the SPs what they believe about the patient they are going to portray can reveal some interesting, and often disparate, attitudes. Here are examples of different responses the SPs initially gave when asked what they thought about the diabetic patient they were all going to portray:

- "This patient doesn't want to get better because he isn't taking his medications."
- "I don't think he knows how sick he really is."
- "He isn't very motivated to give up eating the kinds of foods he's used to. He just likes to party and drink with his friends too much."
- "I think he's ready to make some changes, he just doesn't know how. He needs some specific guidelines."

If attitudes about the patient are not elicited by the coach, they are likely to remain hidden—and every SP will happily assume that everyone else is perceiving the patient in the same way she is. In fact, if an SP's performance is not "on the mark," one of the most fruitful coaching techniques for us to use is to reexplore the SP's attitudes and assumptions about the patient before doing any other kind of coaching.

What are the patient's (character's) expectations about the encounter? The flip side of the coin has to do with what the SPs perceive to be on the *patient's* mind leading up to and during the encounter. This exploration is part of the analytical work that the SPs need to do on their own with the training materials. But, unlike some of their other individual work, the notions the SPs have about the patient they will be portraying *must* be shared collectively. What the patient thinks, is worried about, fears, is convinced of, or expects of the doctor are all important bits of information even if the task of the medical student does not explicitly require him to find out about the patient's frame of mind. The patient's expectations and psychological outlook are valid and central to what she is feeling at the time of the visit and will color her attitude during the encounter. If we and the SPs investigate our own assumptions and the expectations we believe the patient has, it will lead to clarification and a collective mindset regarding the patient's backstory.

Curiosity is the key. Curiosity empowers us to ask questions. It keeps us from being judgmental. It is a quality about which we and the SPs must share a passion. It gets us to the collective answers we need for the SPs to be able to move into the space where the patient "lives" inside each of them.

- What does the patient think is going on with her? What does she think her symptoms mean?
- What does the patient want the doctor to do for him?
- What does she think (or hope) the doctor will tell her?
- What is he afraid to hear or find out? Why? And so on.

Whether the patient's expectations are met and *how* those expectations are handled by the student affects the way the SP feels about the student and the encounter. The secret to unlocking the richness in every patient case is in the effort we collectively make to uncover what is unknown about the patient from what seems obvious. In truth, nothing is obvious. Patients, people, you and I, are complex and contradictory. These aspects need to be brought to light. The analytical work that we do with the SPs naturally leads them to determine what each of them is going to work with, internally, as they perform the case.

The Analysis the SPs Need to Do on Their Own

Once the collective work is done, the SPs need to do their own individual preparation to get ready to perform the case. The actor, William H. Macy, succinctly captured this part of the actor's task in the following three questions (Macy, 2004), which I have adapted for our purposes:

- What is the patient actually doing in the encounter? (This is the part of the collective analysis just described.)
- What is the nature, the essence, behind what the patient is doing in the interaction? (Finding the answer to this question puts the SP in touch with something concrete to "play." (See details which follow under "Working with objectives, intentions, motivations.")
- What is it like for me? (Here is where the actor uses his imagination to make the action personal.)

As part of their analysis, all SPs will find something personal that will help them get in touch with the situation and emotion being experienced by the patient they will be portraying. Why do actors need to do this? Because emotions cannot be played from a cold start. This is not how it works—at least not if the emotion portrayed is to come across as believable. This is why stereotypes do not work. One has to sneak up on an emotion. It has to be coaxed into showing itself. And the ways to do that involve some conscious efforts on the part of the performer. The ways are many, but the goal is the same: The SP's individual analysis of the training materials is meant to guide him toward the internal images that personally mean something to him at the depth that will stir the emotion called for in the patient he will portray.

Said another way, this aspect of the SP's job can be described as finding "that something" that will allow him to enter the world of the patient and start the encounter, or start the acting, if you will. That something goes by different names: the objective, the intention, the motivation. Coming up with that something is integral to the analytical work each SP needs to do.

Right now, all of this may seem to be an abstraction, albeit one that is the responsibility of the actor, the SP. But it is nevertheless an abstraction that, once understood, gives us as coaches a grounding that will help us generically understand how our SPs are shaping their portrayals. These concepts should become clearer as we proceed and will be clearer yet when you have an opportunity to try some of the techniques listed later in this chapter.

Working with objectives, intentions, motivations

[The actor's] job is to communicate the play to the audience, by doing
something like that which the playwright has shown the character to
be doing.

—David Mamet (1997, p. 89)

As we continue our broad exploration of some of the activities that
actors employ to produce their portrayals, working with objectives is
one commonly used acting technique that an SP might use to uncover
the essence behind what is going on inside the patient in order to get
in touch with how the patient feels. In acting, all three of these terms—
objective, motivation, and intention—are commonly used to describe this
same technique. I use all three terms interchangeably as we try to discern
how actors use this tool to prepare to interact in a given situation. For
more detail about any of the acting techniques covered in this chapter, I
recommend *A Practical Handbook for the Actor* written by students of
the playwright/director David Mamet (Bruder et al., 1986) and *Directing
Actors: Creating Memorable Performances for Film and Television* by
Judith Weston (1996).

One of the key results of the SP's individual analysis of the training
materials is the discovery of a personal motivation, which is in keeping
with what the patient is doing/feeling. What the SP is looking for is the
essence *behind* what the patient is doing in the clinical interaction. In other
words, the SP is looking for something he can work with that is in line with
what prompts the patient to act the way he does. This motivation is what
the SP will use to enter into the interaction with the student doctor—
and may use as a touchstone throughout the encounter. By using this
technique, the SP avoids playing a stereotype or an idea about the patient.
The motivation, the objective, or the intention is what the SP will play
when performing the case. He won't play anxiety; he will play "getting
the doctor to tell me my heart is okay." The difference is the distinction
between what the patient-is-feeling and what the SP-is-using to get in
touch with that same feeling. The SP must translate what he understands
is going on inside the patient into something that *he* can do right in the
moment in the interaction. If the SP works with an objective such as
"getting the doctor to order me an MRI" (because the patient is worried
that a tumor might be causing his back pain), the desired emotions of the
patient will emerge. Directly playing emotions are not within an actor's
control. Playing an objective is. Such a technique gives the SP a target to
work toward, instead of trying to play an abstract, amorphous feeling.

It is each SP who will determine the objective he will use. The SP's
personal objective will come out of both his collective and his personal
understandings of the desires and feelings of the patient.

Once again, why are actors doing this? Here is what Judith Weston (1996), who teaches directors how to work with actors, puts it: because "endowing the characters with a need to interact raises the stakes of the relationship" (p. 103)—and, in our case, gives the SP something to hang his feelings on so that he does not become self-indulgent when the emotions he is trying to tap into are stirred. The bottom line is this: *The SP's objective has to do with getting or not getting something the patient wants.*

> A character's objective for a particular scene can be very specific and very simple. For example: I want him to leave the room .... I want him to cry. The simpler it is, the more playable. (Weston, 1996, p. 102)

Notice that this getting or not getting something has both a physical and emotional component built into it. The physical component of the objective is the most obvious. As Weston says, it has to do with

> a win or a loss. To be very simple-minded about it, if my objective is to get someone to leave the room, when he leaves the room, I win; if he doesn't, I lose. In either case our relationship has undergone a small (or a big) change. (Weston, pp. 102–103)

Think about how this physical component of an objective might work for the SP. If I as the SP want the student doctor to give me a prescription, and he does, the relationship I feel with him will express itself quite differently than if he does not. Those specific internal actions are the root of the emotion an actor taps into.

Here's a related concept. The objective is an internal one for the SP who came up with it, but might never be mentioned in the encounter. It is a simple task that *activates* the SP's imagination. If the objective works, it will put the SP in touch with the feeling state needed at the *beginning* of the encounter, and it is what the SP will come back to if his concentration waivers *during* the encounter. It will change the relationship with the student doctor depending on whether or not the objective is accomplished. It boils down to this:

I want something + I get it or I don't get it = I feel something.

Another important notion is that finding an effective objective is about finding something that will bring about an interior *adjustment* for the SP in the immediacy of the encounter. Weston (1996) again:

> It doesn't mean that he [the actor/SP] has any notion that he's going to achieve that objective; it doesn't mean that he's doing anything overt to achieve it. It's his inner life, it gives him an inner point of concentration. (p. 105)

So again, it does not matter what the objective is as long as it helps the SP focus on a need, a want, a desire that creates the internal shift that puts him in touch with the appropriate emotions he is trying to sneak up on.

In fact, the objective need not have anything to do with what is literally going on in the SP's encounter. The objective can actually be something that is surprisingly different from what appears to be going on, such as "I want you (the doctor) to rescue me." Why work with such an intention that in reality is never going to happen? Let's say the patient I am playing is living in an abusive situation, has a negative self-image, is depressed and compliant. These feelings all have to do with being a victim. The SP who comes up with "wanting the doctor to rescue me" is using this intention to tap into those victim feelings. Will such an objective work for every SP portraying this case? No, it will not. Each SP must come up with a motivation that will personally work for her.

Let's summarize what we know at this point. Once the SPs have come to a mutually agreed on understanding of who the patient is, each SP must determine for herself what she wants as the patient, what she hopes to gain from the visit with the student doctor. Is it to get him to order her an MRI? To get the doctor to put his arm around her? To get him to tell her she has a migraine (and not a brain tumor)? This activity is called by several names: finding an objective, a motivation, an intention. It could be something that is out on the table from the beginning of the encounter. Or it might be a hidden agenda that the patient will talk about only under certain circumstances. Then again, it might be something that is never explicitly discussed because it is solely meant to shift the SP's internal environment. The important thing to understand about using this inside-out technique is that it is the SP who must take the shared understanding of the case and make it his or her own; that is, make it something that is personal, that will shift her internal state, and put her in touch with the emotion the patient is experiencing. As coaches we need not know the specifics of the internal process of our SPs as long as they are giving us the performance we are looking for. If, however, the performance is *not* what we are looking for, we do need to explore what the SP is working with and get involved on that level because in these circumstances understanding the SPs' internal process guides us in how to coach their performances.

A few final thoughts about defining objectives: The objective needs to be (a) active, (b) able to be accomplished during the encounter, and (c) positive. In regard to the active quality, Stanislavsky (1999) said that the objective was not to "be expressed in the form of a noun, it must be formulated as a verb..." (p. 193). In fact, this is such an important aspect of creating objectives that there are lists of verbs that have been formulated for actors to use. Continuing with Weston's example of wanting someone to leave the room, here is how the choice of a verb can shift the feeling tone: "If I want you to leave the room, I might *invite* you to leave the room. If that doesn't work, I might *demand* that you leave the room. If that doesn't work I might *beg* you..." (Weston, 1996, p. 103). Can you feel the internal shift between "invite" and "demand" and "beg"? Verbs are synonymous with action—with something that is *do*able. If I, as the SP, want the student doctor to give me an antibiotic, I might reason with her. If that doesn't work, I might flatter her. And if that doesn't work, I might bargain with her.

> If the objective is what the character wants, actions are what he's doing to get what he wants.... Actions are the character's strategy or tactic or approach to obtain the objective.... What they do to overcome their obstacles and to get what they are after are their actions. (Shapiro, 1998, pp. 109–110)

So the actions are in the verbs the actor chooses to work with. This refinement is what gives immediacy, the now-quality, to a performance.

And finally, the most effective objectives are stated in positive, not negative terms. Wanting something is more dynamic than not wanting something. Let's say the SP has chosen "not wanting the doctor to give me a shot" as her intention. Although this objective might be fine analytically, can you see how it is not as playable, not as stimulating as "I want the doctor to prescribe a medication for me"? Wanting something has a forward thrust to it, is more active. Not wanting something implies an absence, is more passive (Cohen, 1978, p. 24).

Before concluding this discussion about objectives, let's look at how an SP playing a patient (who is worried that the chest pain he had earlier means that he has had a heart attack) might define an objective that will support his emotional entry into the encounter with the student doctor. Remember, for the SP it is about (a) What do I want? and (b) How do I get what I want? Here are several examples of motivational statements an SP might use to create an internal shift in playing this patient. The operative word here is internal. These motivations are used to transform the SP's internal landscape. They are not to be played literally as external actions. As you read through the following examples, try to feel the effect— the internal shift—the change that each of the verbs produces inside you:

- I want you to promise me I will be all right, even if I have another bout of chest pain.
  (I'll *press* you to promise me. If that doesn't work, I'll *persuade* you.)
  or

- I want you to give me something to make the chest pain go away for good.
  (I'll *coax* you into giving me something. If that doesn't work, I'll *nag* you.)
  or
- I want you to reassure me that my heart is okay.
  (I'll *plead* with you to reassure me. If that doesn't work, I'll *entrust* myself to you/put myself completely in your hands.)
  or
- I want you to feel sorry for me.
  (If you were the SP, what action verbs might you choose to accomplish an internal shift using this objective?)

To recapitulate, the objective/the intention/the motivation/the action are means of bringing the SP closer to the authentic feeling state of the patient. The ultimate proof of the objective's effectiveness is whether or not it produces the desired emotional results in the SP's performance. If the objective is working, it will help the SP elicit concrete, active images—images from his imagination, fantasy, or memory—that will stir the character's emotion within the SP so that it is available for his use in performance.

Working with the imagination

[The] way to control the emotions needed in a part ... lies through the action of the imagination ....

—Stanislavsky (1999, p. 187)

The use of the imagination is perhaps the most important concept in acting because without a creative imagination, the actor cannot live truthfully under the imaginary circumstances he finds himself in. All along we have been talking about how none of us can *will* an emotion into existence because emotions are the result of "something else" affecting the psyche. That something-else is often beyond our control—someone else's action or something that happens in the external world that affects us. Luckily, there are other ways to get in touch with emotions, ways that *are* under our conscious control. As we have just seen in the previous section, finding a workable objective falls into the frame of action under our control. So, too, can we deliberately and directly summon up images that help us get in touch with feelings.

Images: The royal road to feeling. Mental images are capable of producing the same emotions as actual events. Actors have intuitively known this for a long time, but it has only been within the last decade that scientific research has discovered that the brain processes images and memories in the same way that it processes actual experiences. The brain does not know the difference! This is why working with the imagination is so powerful. As Stanislavsky describes the process, images and fantasy are the way to stimulate "our *affective memory* (emphasis Stanislavsky's, 1999), calling up from its secret depths, beyond the reach of consciousness, elements of already experienced emotions ... and the echo of appropriate feelings," which become naturally available to the actor, without forcing anything (p. 187). So, in essence, actors use images to arouse their memory in order to reconnect to feelings they have previously experienced that are consciously or unconsciously embedded in the image.

Working with the "As If" technique.   Affective memory is one of Stanislavsky's most widely interpreted and diversely practiced ideas. He knew that the actor must have a vivid and creative imagination in order to connect with what the character is supposed to be experiencing. The process of getting to that place for the SP is a progressive transformation starting with an understanding of what the patient is literally doing in the encounter, proceeding to a recognition of the essence *behind* what the patient is literally doing (the objective/what the patient wants), finally leading the SP to uncover in her own imagination what that essence is like for her *personally*. This activity of the imagination can be summed up succinctly in the question and answer: "What's it like for me? It's as if ...."

At this point you might be curious about how the SP links the objective she has chosen to use with the "as if" technique. The SP can use the actual situation of the patient, tap into a personal memory, or create a fantasy. Here is an example: Once the SP has chosen her objective, she might use it to get in touch with her imagination by wholly immersing herself in the patient's actual situation—"as if I were the one being told I have a terminal illness." Not as if the character were being told, but as if *I* were actually being told.

Here is another way an SP might make the connection. Suppose the SP is having trouble putting herself into the patient's *actual* situation. If this is the case, the SP can use her fantasy to bring up images or recall personal circumstances or other memories that cause feelings to arise in her similar to those the patient is having. The SP first asks herself, "What do I, as the patient, want?" (Answer: "I want the doctor to give me a clean bill of health.") However, as the case is written, the student doctor is required to tell the patient that the results of her mammogram have come back positive. So at the point when the student doctor gives her the bad news, the SP uses her imagination to fantasize something that has shock value for her, for instance, "It's as if ... I were being told my mother had been killed in a car accident." Or she could call up a memory of a tragedy she actually experienced in her own life—to get in touch with the emotion needed in the encounter. It matters not whether the SP uses the actual situation of the patient or her own personal fantasies or memories to access the feeling. Actors always end up working, consciously or unconsciously, with images that put them in touch with the emotional/psychological space inside themselves that triggers what the patient is emotionally experiencing at the time of the encounter.

Let's take another example to see how intention and imagination work together. Say I am playing the patient mentioned earlier who is the victim of domestic abuse. The patient's image of herself is so negative that she does not have the wherewithal to take action on her own behalf. She feels imprisoned and does not know how to escape. As the SP, I am working with the intention, "I want you (the student doctor) to rescue me."

How might the "as if" technique be used in conjunction with this objective of wanting the doctor to liberate me from my situation? To raise the stakes of what is going on in the interaction, if I were personally working with this objective of wanting to be rescued and needing to get in touch with the emotional elements of being a victim, I might work with an image that deeply affected me from a story I read of a puppy being stoned to death by a group of angry teenagers. This image holds what I need to be able to tap into the painful feelings required by the case; namely, an identification with a vulnerable, defenseless creature who innocently becomes the object of senseless rage. By activating this image—seeing in my mind's eye the puppy being stoned and her initial attempts to escape—I start to detect the stirring of feelings of confusion, pain, and anxiety within my body. I see the puppy cower and begin to feel her fear, hear her screams, then her whimpering....

If the performer trusts and surrenders to the process while mindfully holding and working with details in an image that is meaningful to him, then the feelings and body sensations hidden in that image *will* naturally emerge for him to use.

Other ways to summon up effective images.   There are other ways to tease out images and thus evoke emotions. Sometimes the perfect image arises from recalling a symphony or a song. Humming the music from the film score of *Schindler's List* is all that might be needed to call forth horrific images of victimization that an SP might use to play an abused patient. Making other kinds of sounds is another way to invite images—often surprising ones. For instance, making the sounds of a whimpering puppy eventually conjured up an unexpected image from a film: one of a Middle Eastern woman, buried upright to her neck in the earth, her head covered with a black cloth, a group of people throwing stones at her head, dying because she was suspected of having done something her abusers disapproved of.

This is how the interconnection of intention and imagination work together to evoke the needed emotion for representing the patient's feeling: The objective provides the SP with a motive ("I want you to rescue me."), giving her something to work with while she is engaged with the student doctor during the encounter. At the same time, the image (e.g., the stoning of the innocent woman in this case) helps the SP get in touch with the emotions (the fear, the pain, the hopelessness) that motivate the abused woman in the patient case to want to be rescued by her doctor.

The willingness of the SP, as an actor, to summon up images—whether they are fantasies of what the patient has been going through or are actual images from the SP's personal memories—puts her in touch with the patient's painful feelings. Using this technique takes courage, as does taking the risk of making a mistake or looking foolish if either the intention or the images do not work for the SP. In using this emotion-evoking acting technique, the SP has to be willing to go there—and stay there—without getting submerged in the emotions that arise as her own feelings. Paradoxical? Yes, indeed—personal, yet not personal—feeling feelings, all the while staying detached enough from them to be able to shape the feelings that arise to fit the requirements of the case. The SP is doing all of this, while at the same time, continually remaining observant of the medical student's behavior and his responses during the clinical encounter. This is the complex and hidden activity that occurs behind every authentic SP portrayal.

Before we move ahead to what goes on in the performance of a case, there is one final, practical consideration. You might be wondering where the SP does this kind of preparation prior to the encounter with the student. The SP usually does the emotional/psychological preparation immediately before the actual encounter right in the room where she will be working—or in any other place where there is privacy and she can be alone to do the necessary work of getting ready for the performance.

Performance of the Patient Case

As you no doubt have surmised, when an actor performs, he lives in multiple realities. An actor can be in imaginary reality at the same time that he is present in actual reality. In other words, he needs to have a foot in, and control over, both worlds. He can release or constrain the internal waves of feeling that have arisen in his body through the creative preparatory work he has done with his imagination. He not only touches the emotion but also rides the waves of that emotion as it is released. Simultaneously, he allows the relevant feelings to prompt his external actions. He allows himself to be played like an instrument. The SP is not in some kind of trance state over which he has no control. In fact, the SP must exercise conscious control over what he is doing all the time so that he can monitor the emotional intensity and choose what he allows to express itself through him. The actor, our SP, knows that the external circumstances in which he is performing are make believe. He is performing out of what that circumstance is like for him. He acts the part as he would if the circumstances were real. He acts "as if" the circumstances *are* real. It is the ability to do this that is the measure of the actor.

Having outlined the substructure of how an actor prepares, we are now ready to look at the elements that are necessary for the performance—the culminating aspect of the actor's process with which we, as coaches, are going to be more directly involved with our SPs. In essence, the performance is the end game that holds in its core all that went before, manifesting all that preparatory work in the present. Once the SP has tapped into the feeling by using the objective and the emotion-evoking images she has chosen, she must have the ability throughout the clinical encounter to *stay present* with both realities, with whatever is going on internally and externally as she plays the part of the patient with the medical student.

Staying in the Moment

An actor in performance needs the ability to stay in the now—in the moment-to-moment unfolding of all that is happening. In order to do this, the SP must be utterly available and responsive to what is going on between her and the medical student in the instant it is happening so that her actions and reactions are relevant to what is going on in the interaction. Living truthfully in the moment-to-moment interactions that take place in the imaginary circumstances of each simulated clinical encounter is what an SP's performance is all about.

So when we talk about *being-in-the-moment*, we are really talking about staying with the ever-changing dynamics of human feelings. This automatically happens when we are living life, but can be disrupted in the artificial milieu of the theater, film, television, and the work of standardized patients. What we are talking about in these imaginary circumstances is the free and natural flow of emotions that the actor must ride throughout the encounter—without letting his extraneous thoughts ("I'm not doing this right" or "I wonder if I got a parking ticket") get in the way of the subtle impulses needing his attention in the moment. Lest you think I am making much ado about nothing—because surely there are times when a person thinks he has no emotions—even boredom and zoning-out are emotional states. Even neutrality is a cover for feelings we are unaware of. We are beings governed by our emotions as much as by our intellects, by our libidos as much as by our cerebral cortex. We swim in the water of feelings all the time. In fact, water is a perfect metaphor for how we live.

Water has profound connections to emotions. What the actor is trying to tap into is "how to let the river of your emotion flow untrammeled, with the words floating on top of it" (Meisner & Longwell, 1987, p. 115).

The point of all the interior preparation an actor does is to help him access that subtle impulse of emotion so that he can play with it as it arises, grows, or diminishes by what is happening between himself and the other. So the emotion can be "ex-pressed" or "re-pressed." So the actor can say one thing and feel another when this is called for. So the SP can focus on the actions and demeanor of the student and shape her own responses by what is true for the patient case she is playing. In essence then, the actor is conscious of what is going on and can make appropriate choices. Here is an example from an SP case requiring the student doctor to give the patient bad news and deal effectively with the patient's response:

> Elaine Andrews must *not* cue the student doctor that she knows she is going to be given an abnormal test result. If she doesn't get a clear enough explanation of the test results, she must ask, "What are you saying? Are you saying that I might have cancer?" This is her "script." Whenever in the encounter this issue arises, she must internally feel the initial shock and disbelief the patient experiences. But because of the way different medical students handle her, she might cry with some of them and not with others. The patient she is portraying might zone out, her mind abuzz with thoughts of disbelief and fear, and be "unable to hear" a thing the student is saying. Or anger might momentarily overwhelm her initial feeling of disbelief.

The details of how the interaction unfolds cannot be predicted. How and when the SP does what she does, says what she says, is dependent on how and when the student does what he does, and says what he says. Our SPs must understand the patient at the core of who she is so that the SP can do her own preparatory work, enabling her to respond authentically in the moment—no matter what comes up.

> The emotion comes with how you're doing what you're doing. If you go from moment to moment, and each moment has a meaning for you, the emotion keeps flowing. I would sum it up by saying that the interpretation is best found in what really moves you. (Meisner & Longwell, 1987, pp. 170–171)

This sounds simple enough, doesn't it? It is—if the actor is able to listen, concentrate, and relax while "playing his part." If the SP cannot do these three things effortlessly, being in-the-moment is anything but simple.

Like everything else we have been exploring in the world of acting—listening, concentration, and relaxation are intertwined elements that are difficult to separate. However, to understand them as an integrated whole, we need to know them, as much as possible, as individual entities that the actor works with in performance. Having a sense of how all these pieces affect the actor's moment-to-moment performance gives us information we need when faced with having to analyze what is causing an SP's performance to go awry.

Listening

To listen is to really take in what the other person is saying, verbally and nonverbally, to the point that it creates a spontaneous response, free of contrivance. When each person in an interaction is really listening, what naturally happens is that each acts and reacts to the other—even when one or both has a particular focus or an agenda. To play off of each other in this way requires presence and concentration—no mind wanderings, no judgments, no self-criticisms to get in the way of what is happening in the moment. Listening is inherent in all good performances. Listening is also an essential skill for the consummate physician. For that matter, so too is it indispensable for us, as SP coaches. Each of us—coach, SP, and student doctor—must be wholly present and focused on the other, ready to adapt instantly to whatever we are consciously or unconsciously perceiving in the other person and in ourselves.

Listening can run the gamut from distraction (actively ignoring) to empathic listening (listening from the other person's point of view). Ideally, the medical student should be working at the empathic-listening end of the spectrum, but, for many reasons, that is often not the case. Therefore, as we work with our SPs, we must be sure they are responding to what is actually happening in the encounter—and not to some idea they might have about how the student *should* be performing. If the SP is able to really focus on the student, he will be able to react appropriately out of the internal impulses that naturally arise to whatever is coming from the student. If the SP is truly listening—not merely biding his time and waiting for his turn to speak—his reactions will be natural, intuitive, and genuine.

For our part, as we interact with our SPs, we also need to listen empathically—listening so intently to what is going on with them that we sense and can respond to what is needed by the specific situation, rather than by imposing an idea about what we think the SP needs or should be doing. This kind of listening (for the SPs and for us) happens in the ever-present silence that exists within each of us—so long as that silence is not disturbed by self-judgment and the fear of being wrong. Access to this silence comes about when we are utterly relaxed, utterly at ease and in the moment. When we are present in this way, we naturally and easily trust that the necessary response will emerge effortlessly when it is needed. Obviously, this is not a state of mind that can be forced (or willed) into being, but just knowing that it exists—and is always there—is sometimes enough of a reminder to bring about the relaxation and ease that allows it to emerge.

Concentration

> .... *creativeness on the stage, whether during the preparation of a part or during its repeated performance, demands complete concentration of all his [the actor's] physical and inner nature* .... (emphasis Stanislavsky's, 1999, p. 186)

This is vintage Stanislavsky. For him, concentration is all encompassing and includes all of the actor's senses. As he says, "it challenges [the actor's] memory, imagination, emotions, reason, will. The actor's entire spiritual and physical nature should be involved in what is happening to the character he has imagined" (p. 186).

On the SP's stage—the clinical exam room—concentration consists of the ability to direct her attention to two spheres. She must be able to focus on the medical student so that she can interact spontaneously in each moment as the interaction progresses. At the same time, she must be able to dispassionately witness what is going on in the encounter so that she can accurately recall what the student said and did when she is filling out the checklist afterward. The way that Stanislavsky visualizes this aspect of the actor's task is in being able to restrict his concentration to within a circle of attention. So, for the SP, this circle of attention not only includes (a) her own feelings, impulses, and responses resulting from intently listening to the student and focusing on what he is doing and saying, but also (b) her witnessing function, which includes observations and her own mental notes of what is going on in the interaction for later use. Here's an example of what can happen if this ability to concentrate in both spheres is *not* present:

> I once worked with an SP who had an uncanny ability to tap into an emotion. She would completely lose herself in the role of the patient (who was being given bad news) to the point that she had no idea what was going on in the encounter. Although her performances were very realistic, her emotional responses were independent of the student's reactions to her. All she needed was a trigger to set off her response to the news, and she did whatever came to her regardless of what the student was doing. Needless to say, during rehearsal she was unable to respond to the variations in how each encounter unfolded, nor was she able to recall the student's behavior, because she was so totally absorbed

in the emotions she was expressing. She literally didn't know what was going on around her.

Although the realism of her emotional reaction was astounding— so much so that those of us working with her found ourselves drawn into the emotion with her—she was obviously not suitable as an SP in either sphere. Her circle of attention had too small a diameter—and the area outside the circle was a black hole.

The necessity of being able to recall the students' behavior makes our SP's moment-to-moment interactions with the students more complex than performing without this requirement. Therein lies the challenge for us, as coaches. We can never forget—no matter how brilliant the performance or how perfect the recall—that our SPs must excel in *both* areas.

Relaxation

For that tiny, invisible inner movement to find its way into the whole being of the actor, "a total relaxation must be there" (Brook, 1968, p. 109). There is no way to access that invisible "flicker" without being utterly relaxed in whatever it is we are doing. Yet there is a natural tendency in all of us to tense up whenever we become anxious or self-conscious. This tension uses an enormous amount of energy, which is wasted as it splits off from where the energy could, and should, be focused. Think about what happens to us in our typical work life. Let's say we are going to give a presentation to a group of people, such as our medical school's curriculum committee. As we think about it, we become anxious, self-focused, our mind spinning around feelings of what our audience will think, or whether they will ask questions that we cannot answer—and we end up wondering whether we are really capable of making the presentation at all. These anxieties are entirely extraneous to our abilities and the goal of our mission, which is to communicate information on a subject we are familiar with. The effect of all this unconscious mental activity, or obsessing, is body tension, which only makes the situation worse. The resulting presentation is often stiff, inflexible, and insulated from the listeners' responses. The speaker's fear of how the presentation will be received has made it rigid and noninteractive.

Realizing that this is what happens gives us a chance to change these circumstances. As soon as we are aware of our anxiety, we need to shift our attention inside, notice what is happening in our body, and become aware of the mental activity that is creating the obstructive internal environment and causing us to tense up. The first step is awareness. Then out of that awareness, we can take conscious steps to work with and alleviate our uneasiness (simply taking several slow, deep breaths is one way of beginning to tame an anxiety response) so that our natural expertise can come through with ease, instead of our being overwhelmed by negative fantasies.

As coaches, we have a similar challenge. We need to create as safe and comfortable an environment as possible so that our SPs can relax and feel secure enough to experiment and discover the patient's feelings within themselves as they work with us in training. The SPs have to feel safe so that they can explore their feelings and not worry about making mistakes, especially in the early part of their training. If they are guarded in what they are doing because they are fearful about what our responses to them will be, their creativity will be stifled. As we have seen, the SPs' fears can come from a lack of confidence in themselves, from the way we are interacting with them, or both. Our SPs need to trust that we will not embarrass them, but that we will tell them the truth about what we are experiencing in their performances. We can also share with them ways to get through their anxiety so that they can work with less tension and more ease.

In conclusion, preparing for performance involves finding an intention to work with throughout the encounter, something the patient wants from the doctor that intensifies the internal involvement of the SP in the interaction. At the same time, the SP, using his imagination, works with an image that is specific and personal to him that puts him in touch with the emotional tone, the feelings of the patient. This combination of intention and image carries the SP into the encounter and supports his performance as he lets go into the moment-by-moment interaction with the student. The SP's responses in the moment are engendered by focusing his attention and listening deeply to what the medical student says and does, all the while remaining mindful and relaxed enough to allow the appropriate, spontaneous responses that emerge from within to express themselves in the encounter. This is the SP's job. Our job, as their coach, is to let the SPs know if what they are doing is working, and to guide them into adjusting their performances when it is not.

CHAPTER SUMMARY

This chapter on acting has

- created the context of the standardized patient case and described the emotional and psychological qualities of the patient that the SP needs to represent.
- established the relationship of standardization of performance with the creative process of portraying the patient.
- shown how analysis of the patient case and knowledge of specific acting techniques can better prepare SP coaches to help their

SPs evoke the spontaneous feelings that produce more realistic performances.
- illustrated the preparation and performance processes the SPs go through to attain the highest levels of authenticity in their portrayals of the patient case.

LOOKING AHEAD

In chapter 4 (Directing: Coaching to Deepen the SPs' Performances), we look more closely at the role of the SP coach as director and how the coach can help the SPs deepen their performances by using the information about acting found in this chapter.

CHAPTER FOUR

Directing: Coaching to Deepen the SPs' Performances

The previous chapter on the art of acting delineated what actors do to create a character, as well as gave examples and intimations of what directors need to know about how actors work in order to skillfully interact with them. That chapter laid the groundwork for understanding what it is that coaches can do to support SPs in their process of coming to an interpretation and performance that fits both with the coach's vision of the clinical encounter and the SPs' understanding of the patients they are portraying.

Putting into words how all of this works is a little like putting the elements of a dance on paper so that the choreography can be studied and repeated by others who have never before seen the dance performed. Keeping in mind that every circumstance, every SP, every coach will need something a little different in order to achieve the same performance goals, what you will find in this chapter is a description of that "dance" between the coach and the SPs, along with a variety of tools and techniques to consider using. It is my hope that by using trial and error and a mixture of techniques that you are drawn to, you will eventually find those that fit and create others that work for you—and that with time these tools will become so integrated into how you coach that you will simply do what is needed. When these skills and techniques have become that much a part of you, you will be able to more completely give in to your instincts and freely follow them no matter what you are faced with. This is the kind of ease we are aiming for in doing our work as SP coaches.

THE RELATIONSHIP OF THE COACH/DIRECTOR
WITH THE SPs

Coaching is the process by which one individual, the coach, creates
enabling relationships with others that make it easier for them to learn.
(Mink, Owen, & Mink, 1993, p. 2)

This enabling process requires the establishment of a relationship
between the SP coach and the individual SPs so that the coach becomes the
SPs' guide, empowering them to grow in their own capacities to produce
realistic performances within the guidelines demanded by the case. In
short, in our role as the coach and director, we need not see ourselves as
authoritarians, but we do need to be clear on what we want from the SPs
in their role of the patient. Our work together is the capstone resting on
the standing stones of acting and directing, balancing the demands of our
own profession within this mutually respectful relationship as we advise
and assist our SPs in preparation for their performances. Because I would
like you to consider working with your SPs in this way, I use the terms
coach and *director* interchangeably throughout this section, because the
SP coach is a director, and the director always needs to be a coach—the
champion and guide empowering the SPs' growth.

As directors, the SPs expect us to know what we want. When we do
not see what we are looking for in an SP's performance, we have to know
what is needed and how to get it. The primary qualities we need to accomplish this are trust that within ourselves we have what is necessary to
guide the SPs in their process—along with a belief that the SPs have within
themselves what we want to see in their performances. That being so, we
need to work with our SPs as partners. We must encourage their intellectual and creative input. We must respect their effort, even though their
contributions will sometimes be wide of the mark and need redirection.

Nevertheless, as we are working collaboratively with the SPs, we
must remember that we are still the final arbiter in our joint efforts. As
one young director said, "I don't want to be a dictator, but I want what I
want" (Shapiro, 1998, p. 217). There's a subtle difference between being
a dictator and being an arbiter. We must believe in ourselves and our
vision. This does not mean that we have to know everything. And, we
can always change our minds when new material helps us see what it is
we are trying to do in a different light. At the same time, we must not
attempt to do the acting *for* our SPs. As obvious as this sounds, what I
mean is that we cannot tell them how to produce an affect, an emotion,
or a reaction. We have to work *with* them. We have to clearly express
what we are looking for and then support them in doing whatever it is
they need to do to realistically deliver what we want. We must invite and

stay open to the risks the SPs need to take as they are discovering who the patient is in their practice encounters during training. This is one of the best ways for us coaches to discover insights about the patient that we might otherwise have completely missed.

It is true that occasionally, like directors in other venues, we do have to decide about make-up for bruises, wounds, scars, and the like, but we have little to worry about in terms of staging or set design, and rarely any costumes other than patient gowns. Aside from vigilance regarding the SPs' factual accuracy in performance and on the checklist, our dominant concern is how to assist them when their portrayals run adrift—or are completely off track. When we are comfortable coaching our SPs' portrayals, the results are unmistakably better, while at the same time, our work becomes more interesting, more challenging, and we have a better time doing what we are doing.

Our job as director starts the minute we are handed a case to train (even before that if we are included in the pretraining phase of case development). As we have seen, this includes everything involved in our own preparation and analysis of the case materials, through working with the SPs to come to a common understanding of the patient, to coaching their performances right up to the last student they work with during an exam.

General Guidelines for Directing SP Performances

If we were to pare down what we need and what we need to do as directors, the list might look something like this:

Know What You Want

Make this your mantra. It is the foundation of everything. How many times have you thought you knew what you wanted only to discover that you really didn't? One way to make explicit to ourselves what we want is to write it down, write it out, tussle with it on paper or on the computer before trying to get it across verbally to the SPs.

Be Straightforward, Honest, Specific, and Objective in Your Feedback to the SPs

Consider these questions that Shapiro (1998) asks of beginning directors:

> Am I afraid of my actors? Am I honest with them? Am I specific, or do I tend to be vague and general? Am I worried about being a nice guy and never really tell them what I think, such as, "Look, you're way off in that scene, and this is the way it should be." Do I think that they

know more about acting than I do and that therefore things will come together for them, when I'm not sure they will? (p. 120)

The SPs expect us to let them know how they are coming across no matter how timid we feel about telling them. Then, if necessary, we must assist them with identifying something (in the circumstances of the patient, in their own life experiences, or in their imaginations) that can help them access the emotional or physical feelings needed for their performances. The more specific we are, the easier it is for the SPs to be specific in their choices.

If you know that something is not quite right, but you are not sure why, it is all right to admit it: "I'm not sure what's going on. I can't quite put my finger on it yet, but something's not quite right. Do you know what I'm talking about?" Often the SP knows that his performance is not working and is uneasy with what he has just done. This kind of invitation opens up the possibility of exploring *with* the SP a hidden insecurity, misconception, or ineffective motivation. Sometimes we just need to think out loud until we discover a way to verbalize what we are sensing in the SP's performance. If we speak with honesty and conviction, the SPs will still be able to maintain the confidence they need to have in us to guide them in doing the work we have hired them to do. There is no need to apologize for not always having a ready fix.

Trust the Process

Use the same techniques in coaching the SPs that actors use in performing:

- Live in the moment.
- Stay focused and listen.
- Be willing to make a mistake.
- Relax.
- Breathe.

Trust Your Instincts

Make friends with the little inklings inside yourself that we often put aside because we do not have words at the ready to express what it is they are saying to us. Then there are the times we take the easy way out because we are afraid of being wrong or afraid of the SPs' reactions. Inklings are good and are often the doorway to something key. If you learn all the techniques in the world and use them in a rigid, lifeless manner, they will yield you lifeless participation from your SPs—and, more than likely, lifeless performances. It is your intuition that makes coaching an art. If we can muster up the courage to think out loud when the inklings are just a whisper, we can begin to understand what it is that needs to shift.

None of this is new, and it is not rocket science, but these principles are a vital part of what all directors do when working with actors. They are pretty easy to understand in the abstract. The challenge comes when we try to put these directives into practice. The good news is that if we work with these elements, the experience will teach us what we need to know. We will learn in the doing. If we have created a safe working environment, the interaction itself becomes a teacher. "Okay, all well and good," you may say, "but what about specifics?"

Other Coaching Principles

Peter Brook (1968) talks about the director being there "to provoke and withdraw until the indefinable stuff begins to flow" (p. 109). That "stuff" is the invisible substance of the play. This is the self-same invisible substance that we and the SPs are working with in our mini-play, the simulated clinical encounter.

Intervene Only When Necessary

Sometimes directors think they need to tinker with actors' performances, otherwise they will not be "acting like a director." Please let go of this notion. It annoys the SPs and causes them to lose confidence in what they are doing.

The truth is, if you are working with SPs skilled in acting, you will have to intervene very little. A simple adjustment in their performance is all that might be needed. You might have to do a bit more work with SPs who have little or no training in acting, but it will probably be a lot less than you imagine. So do not let all the suggestions that follow give you the impression otherwise. It takes a lot of words to describe even the simplest of actions, the simplest step—and we are talking about the dance!

This basic coaching principle of intervening only when necessary runs parallel with the principle of "First, do no harm" that most health care professionals follow when working with their real patients. Do not intervene with your SPs' performance unless it is absolutely necessary—and then only as much as is needed. This is a kind of "doing" by "not doing" approach. In other words, do not get in the way of what the SP is trying to accomplish. Give the SP a chance to discover for himself who the patient is in the situation before interjecting too many suggestions. Training sessions are the place where the SPs should be able to try out for themselves what the patient really "wants" from the encounter and how different "intentions" work with the understanding that each of them has of the patient.

As we work with our SPs to shape their performances, we need to support whatever approach they are using—and not impose another method on them. This does not mean that we cannot make suggestions for them to try. It simply means that where we start is with honoring how they are working. We must give them a chance to experiment with what they have in mind, but not wait so long to intervene that they fail or lose heart. When we have a sense that what the SP is doing is not going to achieve what we are looking for, it is then that we get involved by clearly and simply stating what we want instead.

Sometimes we need to determine whether working separately with an SP outside of the regular training sessions—to help bring her performance in line with what we are looking for—might be effective and worth the effort. Or we may have to recognize whether we are at the point of making the difficult decision that it is time to cut our losses and let the SP go.

Then again, there are many times when we ignore something because we are not sure whether it was what we really wanted. If we are not sure that we have a problem, we cannot even begin to figure out how to fix it. Our job is to experience—from the point of view of the students who will be interacting with them—what the SPs are putting out, then give them feedback on our impressions.

How the SP does what she does and says what she says determines the way the medical student interprets who the patient is. How defines whom. Behavior defines character. As coaches, how the SP's portrayal is coming across to us, how it is affecting us as the stand-in for the student, is the primary material we are working with. This is the stuff to use when suggesting ways to redirect or make adjustments to a performance.

If the portrayal is coming across the way you want it to, the only thing you need to do is let the SP know that you are pleased with what she is doing and cheer her on. It is just as important for the SP to know when you are happy with her performance as when you are not. If you can be as specific about what it is she is doing that pleases you—as you are when her performance is not working—all the better.

Coach By Encouragement

No matter what is going on, no matter how discouraged we might be about what we are seeing in an SP's performance, as coaches it is our job to support and empower our SPs to bring out the best that is in them. After all, we would not have hired them if we had not believed that they were able to do what is necessary. When the going gets tough, it is especially important to remember that our goals and the SPs' goals are the same, and that the SPs' success is our success. Even if our first instinct is to focus on what the SP is doing wrong, it is more productive to shift our initial comments to what *is* working in the SP's performance. This is one very effective way to help the SPs maintain their self-esteem and not become discouraged by negativity—ours or their own.

We need to be continually mindful of creating an environment of encouragement, an environment in which it is safe to take a chance. One way to do this is by holding a positive internal attitude such as, "Look, I hired you. I believe you can do this. I just haven't been able yet to get through to you what is needed." Now, having said this, it does not mean that we must hide the truth as we see it.

Be Candid Without Being Destructive

Do not tell someone their performance was fine if you do not believe it. In other words, do not avoid dealing with areas that need adjustment or redirection. Generally speaking, the SPs know when they are not on, when they are not in the flow, and they also know when we are not telling them the truth. Even though it might be easier to avoid being honest than it is to let the SP know that something is not working, avoiding telling them the truth can erode the relationship we have with our SPs and can create a situation of distrust, not only with the particular SP with whom we are working, but also with the other SPs who are observing the interaction.

By contrast, do not be so harsh in your feedback that you destroy the SPs' courage. It is especially important to let them know what they are doing that pleases you before the first time that you have to tell them that you want them to do something differently. Anyone who has to perform in front of others, no matter how accustomed to it they are, is vulnerable. Exploiting that vulnerability does not work for long—if it ever works at all. There is almost always something the SP has done that deserves positive recognition, even if it amounts to commenting on the SP's good efforts or attempt at doing something you have asked them to try, even if it failed.

One of the simplest ways to frame this attitude of encouragement is to provide them with feedback at regular intervals. In other words, at the beginning, middle, and end of training, let the SPs know what they are do-ing well. In between these assurances, you can comment on anything that still needs improvement. (See chapter 9, Putting It All Together, for more information on how to give feedback.) In the same vein, Judith Weston (1996) talks about using the "language of permission." For example, use "It's okay to do such and such..." rather than "You didn't do so and so." (p. 284). Sometimes all that is necessary is to give the SP permission to do something he is holding back on. Another way to articulate this approach when an SP is not giving you what you are looking for is to first ask him, "What were you trying for in what you just did?" When you understand the SP's perception, you can either work toward your vision (if he is not where you want him to be), or, if his understanding *is* in keeping with your vision, you can proceed with something such as, "Great. That's exactly what I'm looking for, but the way it came across was different from what you intended. What I was experiencing from you was...." Then, if necessary, you can go into more detail on how the SP can deliver what you mutually perceive to be the performance goal. When the SP is finally on the right track, become a cheerleader: "That's it. Now you've got it. Bra-vo!"

When in Doubt, Ask Questions

By asking questions, we invite the SPs to participate. If we always tell them what to do, it not only cuts the SPs out of the process, but it can also cause us to miss possibilities they might come up with that we never thought of. Obviously, we cannot do the acting for our SPs, but we can bring out in them what is needed in the performance by helping them tap into what is already within themselves.

The director must sense where the actor wants to go and what it is he avoids, what blocks he raises to his own intentions. No director injects a performance. At best a director enables an actor to reveal his own performance that he might otherwise have clouded for himself (Brook, 1968, p. 109).

Here are some useful questions to ask the SP:

- What are you working with?
  When we are not getting what we want from the SP's performance, this is the first and one of the most powerful questions we can ask an SP in order to initiate the interaction between us.
- What does this patient want from the doctor?
- Have you ever experienced anything like what the patient is going through?

If you think the problem has to do with a mismatch in interpretation, here are other questions you can ask:

- What do you think is going on with the patient?
- How does the patient feel about being here/about seeing a doctor?

Once you know that the SP's interpretation is in harmony with yours, you can go further:

- What event, what detail in the patient's—or what incident in your own—history holds the essence of that feeling for you?

From answers to these kinds of questions, we are often able to discover what is causing the ineffective performance. We can then follow up with more specific questions, encouragements, and suggestions that will lead the SPs deeper into their own inner resources. Remember, we can mine the backstory details (just as the SPs can) to support them in creating images from which a more authentic performance can arise.

Try to match your style to the needs of the SP when asking questions. Of course, as coaches, we must always tailor the manner in which we ask questions or give feedback based on the personalities and needs of the SPs we are working with and on the relationship we have with them. If I am working with someone who simply needs a wake-up call because her concentration was off and she was merely going through the motions, I might choose to describe what I am seeing in a very direct and blunt manner: "Lillian, it's fake. I don't believe what you're giving me." I can do this because I know Lillian will understand exactly what I mean and know why I am sensing that what she is doing is "fake."

However, if I am working with a shy or timid SP or someone who is not an actor or is insecure in his craft, I will use a different approach: "It's not quite working yet, Randy. You're in the neighborhood, but you don't seem quite connected to what's going on in the encounter (pause for a response.) Are you working with something specific?" What we are trying to do here is to gently uncover something we can use to help the SP go in a direction that will work for him.

For example, let's say we are working with the patient who is worried he has had a heart attack. We want to find something simple and concrete the SP can play. The first thing we need to do is ask ourselves: "What's essential here?" This patient is afraid and unable to put his finger on the fear. Panic is what he's really feeling. He doesn't know what's going on, and he's terrified that he might die! Say this to the SP, then ask, "Have you ever been in a situation where you were panicky—where you felt terrified?" Then see if the SP can come up with some "as ifs."

Actors need something to hang onto, so do not be afraid to give your SPs permission to go over the top or to go with strong choices while you are working with them. If they do not understand what you mean, you might give them an example such as the following as a way to stimulate strong images of their own that they can work with: "You're in an airplane. You feel a jolt—and simultaneously hear a loud bang. You don't know what's happening, but out the window you see flames that you think are coming from one of the engines. You feel the plane bank. There is chaos all around you. You feel like screaming, but you can't. Images flash through your mind . . . ." With something strong to play, the SPs can respond more fully—then you both have something to work with. Do not be afraid of getting too much from the SPs. They can always play with the feelings when there is something available to work with.

Here are questions to ask yourself when analyzing why a performance is "off" or is coming across as fake or overacted:

- Is the actor "trying too hard"?
- Is the SP self-conscious?

If either of these two situations is occurring with the SPs, *you* will feel uncomfortable—and tense. You will feel the tightness coming from them—and in their performances. When something is new or difficult or requires concentration, we tend to tense up and stop breathing "in order to concentrate." But tension blocks the SPs' spontaneity. Our job is to help them reestablish movement so that they can relax into the flow of what is happening in the interaction. Instructing the SPs to relax is usually ineffective, but reminding them to breathe is one simple, effective means of bringing awareness (without judgment) to the tension that is getting in the SPs' way.

Simply take a time-out with the SP and ask her to breathe. Encourage her to inhale slowly through her nose until her lungs are filled with air, hold for a count of seven, then exhale slowly through a slightly opened mouth until all the air is gone. Have the SP do this several times while focusing on her breathing. (By the way, this works for anyone who is feeling tense—the SPs, the students, us—under any circumstances.) Breathing in this conscious way works on a physiological level as well as on a psychological one and refocuses the mind away from the incessant, inner destructive chatter that says, "This isn't working. I'm not doing this right. I'm the only one that's not getting it . . . ." Once you have worked with an SP in this way, all you might need to do in the future is remind her, "Breathe . . . ." Then when she is ready to go back into the encounter, you can encourage her with something like "Okay, now, make it simple. Just talk to me."

What if self-consciousness or trying too hard are not the SP's issues and we are not sure why the performance is coming across as phony? If this is the case, we obviously need to investigate further. Here is the beginning of an actual dialogue in a training session as the coach starts to explore what is behind an SP's overacted performance.

Coach: What are you working with, Emily?
SP: What do you mean?

Coach: What do you want from the doctor? (Pause for response)
What's your motivation in coming to the clinic today?
SP: I'm trying to be Maria [the name of the patient].
Coach: And what is that? I'm not sure what you mean.
SP: I'm trying to become Maria. I'm trying to express what
she feels....

This interaction highlights a common mistake made by actors and non-actors alike. When the SPs are "trying to be the patient," they're sure to fail because they can't *be* the patient. It is impossible. No one can be someone else. No actor can become the patient. The patient is a fiction, a person only in the SP's imagination. Therefore, anything the SP does in trying to be the patient is going to be false. The truth exists in making the patient's *situation* her own. It's a subtle difference, but an important one. The SP is *not* the patient. The SP is *speaking for* the patient.

Specific Ways to Assist the SPs

The following ideas might help you further explore the patient portrayal with the SP.

Playing the Situation

Whenever we discover, as in the previous example, that the SP is trying to *be* the patient, our job is to help the SP shift into playing the situation—into playing the given circumstances the patient finds himself in (all of which should be laid out clearly in the training materials). Our job is to guide him into playing something simple and concrete—for instance, into playing what the patient wants from the doctor. Playing a believable action on behalf of the patient will cause an effect in the SP. It will activate the SP's imagination, which in turn will cause something to happen to him internally—he will organically start to feel something.

Focusing on the Other

At this point we may find ourselves at another juncture where a performance can get derailed and, therefore, at another place where we might need to intervene. The SP must be able to stay with whatever feeling is activated internally and, at the same time, focus on the student and what is coming from her—the words she is saying, her tone of voice, her actions—and how all of that is affecting him in the role of the patient. In other words, in order to stay in the moment with whatever is going on in the interaction, the SP has to be at home in both places. He has to be of two minds, so to speak. If we can help him relax into this dual focus, it will become the launching pad for entering the flow of feelings that are engendered while the interaction is unfolding.

Remember, too, if the process is alive for the SPs, throughout training they are constantly asking themselves questions about the patient they are playing. Indeed, these questions are part of their image making. So, do not feel that you have to have an answer to every question they ask you. In fact, sometimes the most effective thing you can do is repeat the question back to *them*, especially if you get a sense that the SP has the answer and only needs to dig a little deeper: "Why *did* he wait so long to call an ambulance when he got the chest pain this morning?" Or simply, "What do *you* think?" Even when you do have an answer, this is often the best route to take. If you let the SP discover the answer, it means more because he will have found his own way to the source of feeling.

Helping the SPs Reproduce Realistic Physical Pain

Pain is the most common physical finding the SPs are required to reproduce. Before we can help them bring to life the specific pain described in the training materials, it is helpful to look at what pain consists of from the standpoint of coaching. Pain is an internal, physical sensation accompanied by an emotional response that often makes itself known in some kind of external manifestation—the inability to move in a normal fashion, tensions in various places of the body, protection of the place where the pain is most intense, facial expressions, vocalizations, manner of speaking, tone of voice, and so on.

There are many ways to approach working with an SP who is having trouble simulating a realistic portrayal of physical pain. What follows are three examples. The first is a technique from Stella Adler, a teacher of acting who studied directly with Stanislavsky and who, over the course of time, through her own students, has had a powerful influence on the whole field of acting. The exercise I have chosen is one in which Adler uses the "as if" technique to help an actor express the pain of a migraine headache. Following Adler's exercise, there are two other examples of ways to coach the reproduction of pain—one starting from the inside, the other using specific physical actions to elicit the desired feelings.

Once again, these techniques are offered here mainly to inspire you to use your own creativity when working with your SPs.

Exercise Using the "As If" Technique

As we have seen, one way that SPs can reproduce emotion is to conjure up a personal memory. This method works equally well with producing realistic physical pain. The SPs can use a personal memory—a sense memory—of a pain similar to the one the patient is experiencing. We will look at that method in more detail in a moment in the second exercise. In Stella Adler's approach, the imagination is used in different ways to conjure up images that are equally powerful but are *not* part of the SP's personal experience. Adler's technique can be particularly helpful to use with SPs who cannot reproduce, or have not themselves experienced, the kind of pain the patient is living with.

As you read through Adler's images, try working with this technique yourself. Pick the suggestion that is most potent for you, close your eyes, and use your imagination to create that image, that imagined action. *Do not try to produce a reaction.* Simply *allow* whatever reaction comes up, to play itself out. Imagine the headache "as if"

1. Someone were pushing in your eyeballs.
2. You were making a hole in your eyes.
3. I were sticking a needle into your eye.
4. I were pouring strong alcohol into it to clean it. (Adler, 1988, p. 45)

Which parts of your body were affected by working with your chosen image? Were you surprised that you felt reactions in places in your body other than in your face? Where in your body did you feel tension or aversion? Once the SP has come up with an effective image (one of her own or one through your encouragement), she must be able, in a relaxed way, to focus on the image and allow whatever arises to manifest itself in her body. She must not anticipate, or work at producing, a reaction to the image. Instead, she must use the image as a trigger for the reaction. Then, as Adler (1988) says, "The imagination awakened by the 'as if' will give you a technique to experience pain in any part of your body" (p. 45).

Now let's look at two other ways of assisting your SPs in producing believable physical simulations. We start with working from the inside-out.

Exercise Using the "Inside-Out" Method

Let's say the pain is one associated with a perforated ulcer. The entire abdomen is affected and the pain is excruciating, especially if the patient moves or her abdomen is touched. If the SP has ever had a similar kind of pain, an obvious first step is to suggest that she use this experience to re-create the pain in her imagination. But what if the SP has never had excruciating belly pain before? Ask her if she has ever had any other kind of severe pain that she might use as a doorway to slip through into the experience of this type of ulcer pain. Let's say she has had extremely painful menstrual cramps or abdominal pain from food poisoning. Or it could have been an excruciating pain that the SP has experienced in some other part of her body such as a broken bone, a dislocation, an earache, or a toothache.

The first task is to encourage the SP to focus on the area of the original pain. Remind her to concentrate on remembering details of what the pain felt like. Was it one solid block of pain? Or were there nuances of sensation—an underlying ache with sharp stabbing pain coming periodically in waves? Ask her to focus on that solid block and allow her body to respond in any way it wants to when she feels the sharp, intense pain—as she will have to do when she moves around on the exam table or when the medical student touches her abdomen.

If you are still not getting what you are looking for, you might want to ask her to imagine—as Adler has suggested—each sharp pain as if someone were stabbing her in the stomach with a knife. Bring into play whatever works.

Exercise Using Specific Physical Actions

Continuing to work with the patient's symptoms of a perforated ulcer, let's say that even the image of being stabbed in the stomach is not working for your SP. It could be that she is so self-conscious she cannot focus one-pointedly enough or perhaps she is untrained and has never worked in this way before. Whatever the reason, there is yet another way to work with your SP. Now is the time to suggest conscious physical actions that can ease her into working with her imagination and help her to focus, go inside herself, and enter into an image that has emerged out of the physical work. Remember most often this kind of exercise is best done in a private session with an SP who you feel might benefit from this way of working. When we work with this technique, our goal is to guide the SPs in using their bodies as a means of stimulating images and internal feeling responses connected with the physical actions we are asking them to perform. This needs to be our mindset throughout the coaching during this exercise (whether we tell the SPs specifically what it is that we are doing before we start the work with them or in the midst of the process).

Now ask the SP to tense up her abdominal muscles as if someone is about to punch her in the stomach—and hold that tension as if she is protecting herself from the pain that such a blow would induce. Then ask her to relax the rest of her body while continuing to hold the tension in her abdomen. See what she does. The relaxation you are looking for is an emotional/psychic relaxation, but it can be induced by asking the SP to relax another part of her body (for example, her shoulders while she is still holding the tension in her belly). Watch what happens to her breathing. She should not be able to take a normal breath at this point. Ask her to take a little breath against the abdominal tension and let out a sound as she exhales without opening her mouth. Ask her to try to take her mind off of the pain by counting the waves as a way to make the "pain she is feeling" less severe. This counterbalancing of energies serves two purposes: (a) it gives the SP something active to do within the imagined pain and (b) it helps her concentrate on the details (the sensations) of the pain by involving her in the activity of counting.

Once she has gotten this, ask her to hold back and not make the sound that she "wants" to make. And so on. You get the idea. You encourage the SP to play the opposites—the tension and the relaxation, the giving and the receiving, the feeling and the resistance to feeling. Eventually, something should happen—some images, some memories should emerge—in the "doing." The key thing to remember is that in order for this to work, the SP must trust you and be fearless in following where you are taking her. Otherwise, she will protect herself from getting in touch with the genuine reactions that must be allowed to surface if her performance is to ring true.

Keep this intense coaching up with the SP until you sense she is getting it and producing what you are looking for. Having taken her through this experience, you will have demonstrated to the SP how she, on her own, can work with physical actions and the memories and images they induce. If she is wholly concentrated on re-entering that imaginary reality, her body, her affect, her voice will naturally reflect the pain she is re-creating.

After this kind of coaching, the SP will need to practice many times on her own so that during the next training session she can hold the imaginary reality at the same time she is producing the actual physical findings—such as the meticulously careful, slow move from being on her side to lying on her back, the abdominal guarding, the intense response to palpation.

Finally, all SPs must be able to stay with the appropriate amount of pain *throughout* the encounter. If the SP cannot maintain the pain affect, of course the realism of the performance will suffer, even if she can faithfully reproduce the specific physical features of the medical condition. In short, whether the image the SP is using is derived from a previous personal experience of pain or not is less important than (a) how effectively the SP assimilates the imaginary sensation she is using and (b) how capable she is of allowing her body to manifest, throughout the duration of the interaction, the appropriate physical and emotional reactions that are stirred once that process has been initiated.

Helping the SPs Adjust Their Performances

> One thing is clear to me: there are directors of the result and directors of the root. We must distinguish one from the other. We need directors of the *root*.
>
> —Stanislavsky (Cole & Chinoy, 1986, p. 109)

When a performance is not coming across as we have conceived it, the most common instinct is to show and tell the SP how to do it right. For instance, if the SP is not acting angry enough, we may take the last line he said in the interview and repeat it back to him in an effort to demonstrate the inflection and tone of voice we want him to use. Or we may simply say such things as, "You're not depressed enough," or "I need you to be more anxious." It's all the same. We're asking for a *result*. This is not the most effective way to get what we want, however.

In essence, by doing this, we are asking the SP to imitate us or to jump to the final outcome without our supporting the work they must do to get there. When they need help, what they really need from us is assistance in finding a way to shift their internal process so that they can give us the performance we want. We usually fall into the do-what-I-do, can-you-try-something-different, or bring-it-up-a-notch mode because we are frustrated at not seeing in their performance what we had in mind. We are frustrated at not being able to communicate with the SPs so that they understand the meaning rooted in our request for more or for less. This is what we naturally fall back on when we are tired or looking for an easy fix. And, truthfully, sometimes it works, but not because of the specific reading we have given the actor. If it works, it is more likely that the SP was able to discern the intention behind the result direction we gave, then used that information to inform her subsequent performance.

Look at it this way: Trying to fix the problem by focusing on the result would be like a physician giving her patient (whom she wants to be pain free) a narcotic, without discovering and treating the root cause of the pain. If she only treats the symptom, to get the result she wants (freedom from pain), and not the cause of the pain, the pain is going to come back as soon as the medication is stopped. If we only deal with the result we want in the SP's portrayal, her performance is likely not going to be affected in the way we would like. *What* are we really trying to communicate when we say, "It looks good, but I need you to be angrier"? *That's* the question we need to ask ourselves. Until we can get to the root of what we are looking for in the SP's performance, more than likely we won't get what we want—and not because the SPs won't try to be angrier. They will.

Communicating in the Language of Images

In order to help the SPs give us what we really want, we have to speak the language they speak. We have to communicate with them in words and ideas that produce images. Here is where having even a little bit of understanding of how actors do what they do comes to our aid. For the SP to accomplish the result we want, he has to consciously or unconsciously go through that image-evoking process.

If the SP is having trouble, it is our job to support him in finding the images that will produce the internal shift that needs to take place. Finding that internal shift has nothing to do with the rational mind, with intellectual discussions about the patient or explanations of how the patient would or would not act. The internal shift happens by using the imagination. When something shifts internally for the SP, there is a physical sensation that accompanies the shift because, as we know, even though emotions are triggered in the brain, they are also experienced in the body. The body, the mind, images, and emotions are all interconnected. This is why working with body sensations can produce images, memories, feelings—and the performance we want. Tapping into one can bring to life any of the others. Any one of them can coax feelings into being. So if the performance is not working, *what actors need from directors is help in finding an image that works.* Likewise, this is what our SPs are looking for from us as their coaches.

So, let's briefly look at a few ways to stir an actor's imagination. It could be a memory of an event in the SP's own life, a phrase, a symbol, a song, a fantasy, or something in the circumstances of the patient that will help the SP get in touch with the feeling, the emotion that is needed. Here are a few examples of working with such image-evokers:

1. This is an exchange between a coach and an SP playing a tight-lipped adolescent being forced by her mother to come to the clinic for her annual check-up:

   > Coach: I'm not sure what's going on, but it feels as if you're challenging everything the student is saying.
   > SP: Yeah, well, the patient doesn't want to be here.
   > Coach: Right . . . but you're not mad at the student. The student didn't do or say anything to upset you . . . .
   > SP: (Silence)
   > Coach: What if you had a fight with your mother just before she dropped you off at the clinic?

   With the question hanging in the air, let the SP come up with her own image of that event. If she needs more, you might encourage her with: "Can you remember the last time your mother made you do something you didn't want to do?"

2. The SP is portraying a patient who is the victim of domestic abuse. Her performance is lacking a sense of the vulnerability and fear the patient is living with. So instead of asking her to be more vulnerable, you invent some backstory on the patient:

   What if your boyfriend has just beat up your two small children's pet cat and is now threatening to harm them: "The next time you or your brats get out of line I'm going to beat the crap out of the lot of you."

3. The SP is playing a patient who is skeptical of doctors, but she has been having chest pain and feels the need to get it checked out. The patient's misgivings about putting her trust in the hands of the doctor are not coming across. You suggest:

   The last doctor this patient saw rushed through the physical exam, literally tearing the paper gown off her as he proceeded....

4. The SP, playing a patient who is afraid that his new doctor will be reluctant to fill his narcotic prescription, is not getting this feeling across. You encourage the SP to flatter the doctor:

   What if you were to (internally) fawn all over everything that comes out of the student doctor's mouth?

5. You can invite the SP to

   - silently hum a piece of music (that holds the appropriate feeling for him).
   - recite to herself a phrase or a fact from the training materials that captures the essence of the patient for her.
   - repeat a line from a poem until "something happens."
   - repeat an exclamation or phrase that holds the emotion he is looking for ("Oh shit!" or "Yeah, right...." or "Oh, my God!" or "Whatever...." or "I gotta get outa here.") again and again until a memory, an image, or a feeling—a flicker—emerges.

Guiding the SPs in Discovering and Working With Their Chosen Images

Once the SP has come up with an image, either on her own or with assistance from you, it may still be necessary to coach her in actually working with that image. This is especially common when working with SPs who do not have a background in acting, but it is occasionally useful even when directing actors.

Remember, images are made up of details, and the feeling is stored in those details. Therefore, trying to coax a feeling out of a nonspecific image or vaguely remembered experience will not work because the feeling resides in the particulars. Knowing this, you can encourage a struggling SP to explore the details in the image he is working with. If necessary, you can even guide the SP on his internal exploration. Tell the SP there is no need for him to verbally answer the questions or prompts you suggest. Be sure to give him time to follow where you are leading him:

> Where are you? What do you see in your surroundings? Be specific. What's drawing your attention? Is there anyone else there with you? Where are they in relation to you? What are they/you wearing? Is there any particular smell you notice? What about sounds? And so on....

When a feeling arises, ask the SP what detail he has just discovered. That's the "particular" that is holding the feeling he is experiencing. It is that detail he can use as the touchstone when he needs that feeling in the encounter with the student. You can coach the SP in this way, even without knowing what he is actually working with—giving him the privacy to work with something very personal.

I continue to be amazed at how often SPs have been cast to play patient cases that have sensitive elements similar to those they have experienced in their own lives, without any of us, including the SPs, knowing this when they were recruited. Therefore, as we accompany the SPs, this work has to be done with the utmost respect for their willingness to revisit experiences—painful or not—in their own lives. Although using a powerful, personal memory is sometimes the ideal choice for an SP, keep in mind that sometimes those memories are still too raw for the SP to work with effectively. Unless enough healing has taken place around the experience, the emotions that surface will not be within the SP's control. The performance could then become about the SP working out his own unresolved issues, instead of about tapping into an emotion he has control over—an emotion that is part of the built-in challenge of the case for the students. We must continuously have our feelers out to detect when the SP might be unconsciously going into territory that he is not yet ready to utilize in this way.

If you sense that this might be the case, the first thing to do is let the SP know: "You seem to be using pretty powerful stuff here...." Wait for a response, then ask the SP what he thinks about what you have observed. If you sense from the SP's response that he does have control over the emotion, you can continue to work with him on it. If, however, you feel he is working with material that has the potential to overwhelm him, you can give him permission to not go there, for example: "It's okay to use something else if this image is too much to work with right now." Having said all of this, truth be told, this kind of situation does not come up every day, but it does happen enough (especially with SPs who are just learning to work with images) that it is useful to know what to look for and how to approach the SP when it arises.

Here is an example of a coaching technique that involves having the SP place in her body the image of the experience she is working with. Have the SP decide where the image would like to reside in her body. Suggest that she sit quietly with the image, then let her know that the image may stay or go elsewhere in the body if it wishes. Encourage the SP to let her body generate whatever emotion wants to emerge from the place where the image is resting. The following illustrates one way to work with this technique. It occurred during a private coaching session I had with one of the SPs who had been hired to play the Maria Gomez case (the sample case in Appendix A):

> During the first training session, this particular SP produced such an artificial, over-the-top reaction to the news that she might be pregnant, there was no question that some coaching was needed. After working with her for a bit, I realized the need for a separate meeting with her. I didn't know exactly what I was going to do, but I knew if I couldn't coach her into a better performance, we would have to face letting her go. After the training session, I mentioned that I wanted to work with her to see if together we could come closer to the truth of what this young patient was going through. (As you know, part of the backstory on Maria is that she is still living at home and is close to her deeply religious parents who do not like her boyfriend and are adamant that she not have sex until she is married.) This is how the early part of our private session unfolded. I started with "What do you think this patient wants from this visit to the doctor?"

> SP: Probably something for the abdominal pain, I guess....
> Coach: Do you have any sense of what it might be like for this patient to be told she might be pregnant instead of getting something to take the pain away?
> SP: (Silence)
> Coach: I wonder how it might be for you if you yourself thought you might be pregnant?

> At this point, I was simply beginning to explore options in hopes of finding something the SP could relate to, something she could fantasize about to help her get in touch with the emotion that was needed to portray this patient. To my surprise, the SP volunteered that in the previous year she had in fact been in a situation like the one Maria was in. She had jumped right in to where we needed to go—to something she might be able to work with that could put her in touch with what the patient was experiencing.

I was getting a sense that this SP's overacting had been due both to her lack of acting experience and to her not wanting to get too emotionally close to what had personally been a very difficult situation. After assessing where she was emotionally in terms of working through her own painful feelings, we both felt comfortable with having her try to access that experience while we were working together—to determine if it could be used to produce a more believable performance, or to decide if we needed to find another means to access the appropriate feeling.

I asked the SP if she was willing to try an exercise with me, assuring her that she could stop at any time. I shared with her that I was going to ask her to close her eyes and put the memory of her own experience into her body, more specifically into her belly and let it sit there. I told her I was not expecting her to do anything or say anything in particular. All I wanted was for her to stay with the feeling and "see what happens—and if nothing happens," that was all right too.

We sat in silence for several minutes. I watched her, looking intensely for any external signs that might give me a clue about her inner experience. There was no change in the SP's body language or demeanor, so I asked her if she could share what was going through her mind. She began by telling me she was thinking about her brother and how he would have been so disappointed in her if she had actually been pregnant. As she started to veer off on a story, I encouraged her to "stay with the feeling." After a bit more silence, I asked, "Where is the feeling now?" "It's still in my stomach." "Okay, what's it like?" As she started to describe it, she stopped—and then began to cry silently. "Are you all right?" I asked. "I'm fine. I'm just thinking about how the guy didn't even really care about me, how used I was; how if I had been pregnant, how he would not have been there for me—how stupid I was . . . ."

She was still crying. "Are you all right with this?" I asked. "I'm fine," she said. "Okay, can you hold this feeling and try to do a part of the interview with me?" She nodded—and so we did the part of the interview where the patient finds out that indeed she might be pregnant. The SP's performance was just right. She felt it—and so did I. She needed no further coaching during this session.

At this point in the coaching it is important to make explicit what the SP is going to have to do to be able to produce the feeling again in the future. The SP needs to know what to expect, what you want, what is involved, and what she is working toward. When this SP came out of the "interview," we talked about how the experience felt for her—how it felt to be using her own real experience to access the body sensations to gain entry to the emotions that would make up her performance. Before she left, we also talked about how she might access this place inside herself, not just once but multiple times during an exam administration, how much discipline it was going to take to be able to accomplish this kind of consistency, and how challenging it might be for her to maintain it.

Going With Your Gut

Even if you are not sure of what you are doing as a coach, if you respond in the moment and get beyond the thoughts that are creating the fear of inadequacy we all experience periodically when we are pushing our edge, you will actually find that there is some place inside you that does know what you are doing. This fear is usually most potent when something is new. Going with your gut simply means trusting your instincts and feelings—including being open to letting the SPs teach you what you need to know.

Creating the Same Challenge

Even though the following example does not have to do with coaching SPs on their emotional performance, it does have to do with another equally important aspect of coaching—making sure that the SPs are creating the same, appropriate challenge for all medical students who will be taking the exam. Like everything else having to do with coaching, this part of training also requires us to use our instincts.

One SP, let's call her Margaret, venerated as the grande dame in our local acting community—and someone who so intimidated me by her reputation that I almost didn't hire her—during training played an older patient in a brilliant, but repeatedly unacceptable manner. The patient she was portraying is a 72-year-old woman who is living alone and generally views her appointments with the doctor as social visits, talking up a storm about everything that comes into her mind. However, at this clinic visit she was also "a little worried" because she had been feeling "woozy." Margaret played the endearing affect of this patient perfectly, improvising details in her chatter that were realistic, poignant, and amusing.

The problem was that she was too good at being chatty. She intuitively knew how to keep the stream of consciousness going. She would start a new topic before quite finishing the previous one, leaving no gap, and making it inordinately difficult to interject, validate, or interact with her verbally. What she was doing in her performance was making the challenge for the student doctor too difficult. During training, I tried various ways to coach her into giving me some space to interact with her, saying, "I feel frustrated because I can't find any way to interact with you other than to nod my head. As the student doctor, I need to be able to ask you questions and respond to what you are telling me without having to cut you off." We tried it again several times, each time thinking I had gotten through to her. Finally, when I was working with her during the last round of interviews with everybody, without thinking about it, I stopped the interaction and said firmly, "Zip it up, Margaret." She flashed back, "You're stifling my creativity." And again, before I could think about it, I heard myself say, "No, I'm not, I'm containing it. In fact, this challenges you to be creative in a different way." To my surprise, she smiled. She knew this venue was not about showing off her acting talents. She knew this was about working with novices and creating for them the appropriate challenge for their level of learning. She knew her job was to give them a chance to demonstrate their ability to interact with a talkative patient and *still* be able to work up a medically difficult case in a relatively short period of time. By the beginning of the exam, all I had to do was the zip-it-up gesture across my lips to remind her. Eventually, when she would see me coming she would do the gesture before I could. It was then that we both knew we were where we needed to be.

In Conclusion

So here we are as coaches about to walk out the other side of the portal created by the Stones of the Dolmen. But before we move on to the work of recruiting, auditioning, selecting, and training, let's reflect on some of the things we have explored about acting and directing to enable you to become a more effective SP coach.

- Become a standardized patient. There is nothing like firsthand experience to give a perspective of the other side.
- Take a class in acting and/or directing.
- Listen to your SPs. Try to hear with your eyes, see with all your senses—go beyond the words.
- Help the SPs get beyond fear and self-judgment. Help yourself, too.
- Do no harm. Intervene only with the SP when you are not getting what you want.
- Help the SPs find "a strong, playable action." Use verbs. Verbs are inherently active.
- Watch out for result direction. It is not your job to get the actor to behave in a *specific,* set way.
- Speak to the SPs in the language of images. It is all about images that mean something to the SP. It is all about helping them find those images to tap into an emotion.
- Be honest, simple, and concrete. Don't blather. Encourage the same from your SPs.
- Allow the SPs to do the work. Do not do it for them. Remember Brook's counsel of "provoke and withdraw."
- Stay present—and help the SPs to stay in the moment, too.
- Encourage the SPs to focus on what is going on with each student and play off of their reactions.

- Follow your instincts and help the SPs follow theirs.
- Use the body to help the SPs make the internal shift needed. Remember the exercises to induce anxiety and anger. Create others of your own. Ask the SPs what they do to entice these emotions into being.
- Let the SPs know when you are pleased.
- Relax. Breathe.

CHAPTER SUMMARY

This chapter has

- described the advantages of a collaborative relationship between the coach and standardized patients.
- provided guidelines for directing the SPs' performances.
- discussed such principles of coaching as minimal intervention, encouragement, and being candid with the SPs.
- suggested specific ways to help the SPs to portray a patient's pain and emotion and to fine tune their performances.

LOOKING AHEAD

Now that you have more of a sense of how to evoke deeper, more nuanced performances from your SPs, through the application of acting and directing skills, I want to share some of the finer points of recruitment and training. The chapters in Part Two explore these topics in depth. We start in chapter 5 with Casting: Finding the Right Standardized Patients. The succeeding chapters give detailed descriptions of the training sessions and the procedures you can use to prepare standardized patients to perform in any high-stakes clinical skills assessment.

Training Procedures: Casting and Training the Standardized Patients

CHAPTER FIVE

Casting: Finding the Right Standardized Patients

Finding the right person to portray a particular patient is as crucial to the ultimate success of the case as are the quality and completeness of the materials written for this purpose and your skill as an SP coach. Together these three elements form the foundation for the quality and the authenticity of the standardized patient experience. This chapter is devoted to recruitment, auditioning, and selection—procedures that will help you find the best people to play the various SP cases in your clinical exam[1] and those who are also best able to take direction from you.

RECRUITMENT

The way we find and train our standardized patients should be handled in the same spirit, with the same high standards of quality, and with the same sensitivity that we expect the SPs to exhibit in all of their activities with the faculty and medical students as they become part of the larger teaching mission of the medical school curriculum. We standardized patient educators and our SPs should be working toward making the process of learning more experiential, more humane, more relational, more like

---

[1] Prior to recruiting, you should have already set the dates for the "mock" Practice Exam and the administrations of the CPX. There should be a minimum of two days between the Practice Exam and the start of the CPX to allow enough lead time to refine administrative procedures, work on details with the SPs and staff, and take care of any other matters that were identified as needing attention during the Practice Exam.

the ideal of what the practice of medicine can be, both for the physician and the patient.

Recruitment Principles

Using the following principles should help you locate the most appropriate individuals to audition for the patient cases you are casting.

Recruit SPs Whose Profiles Are as Close to the Case Descriptions as Possible

As obvious as this seems, it is important from the beginning to bring in only persons who fit the demographic description of the case. When you find yourself in the situation of not being able to recruit enough people with the specified characteristics (which is not uncommon), it is important to formally consider extending and/or changing the demographic requirements.

Before deciding to modify the patient characteristics, check with the case author or your CPX advisory committee[2] to determine whether such a change in demographics might have an adverse impact on the intent of the case, or might affect the way a student approaches the challenge of the case and thus influence the data collected.

Stay Open to the Possibilities. Remain Flexible. Be Willing to Change Your Mind

The demographics on most cases have some leeway. There have been occasions when decisions have been made to expand the demographics of a case for reasons other than difficulty in recruitment. It is common for a person to be called in to audition for a specific case, and during the audition be asked to read for one or more other cases for which they may also appear suitable. Ethnicity, age, and gender are the three main demographics to consider when recruiting. More research is needed to

---

[2] The responsibility of the CPX advisory committee is to maintain the high standards that make the Clinical Practice Examination a reliable measure of the examinee's clinical competence. Members of the committee may include clinical faculty, the CPX psychometrician and/or statistician, and the SP coach. On an as needed basis, this committee may be asked to review the video recordings and checklists of any SP whose performance progress is in question during training. This committee may also be responsible for determining pass/fail cuts and honors from the data analysis on the exam, as well as which students require clinical skills remediation.

determine the potential effect that these factors might have on SP accuracy in both performance and checklist recording, but in the meantime, here are some things to think about in each of these areas when casting for your exam.

Ethnicity

Decisions about changing the ethnicity of a patient are always case dependent, as illustrated in this example:

> Recently, when auditioning a woman who was not already in our patient pool, it became clear as we worked with her that she naturally had the qualities we were looking for in a different case. This woman possessed an underlying sense of vulnerability that she was attempting to cover up with a kind of worldly confidence—qualities that were characteristic for a case in which the patient was to be given unexpected bad news during a routine follow-up clinic visit. The demographics of this case called for a Caucasian woman, but during the audition, this African American woman's ability to portray the devastation of a woman newly being told she might have a terminal illness was so convincing that we decided to explore expanding the ethnicity of the case in order to include this woman as one of the SPs. It seemed we had an opportunity to work with an exceptional performer who, already, in the audition, was giving a powerfully realistic portrayal of the case.
>
> The physician director of the CPX advisory committee and the psychometrician for the exam were consulted and the decision was made to allow the African American woman to play this patient, because ethnicity did not appear to have an impact on the objectives of the case. As part of this decision, we also did an informal study of whether the students performed better or worse with the Caucasians or the African American woman. The results of our data showed that our intuitions were correct: In this particular case, the change in ethnicity did not affect the challenge of the case for the students (giving bad news and dealing with the patient's response) and, therefore, did not adversely impact how the students performed on this case.

Age

The age range on most cases can be extended without detriment to the case objectives. However, for standardization of physical characteristics, it is still important to try to hire all SPs who look to be no more than a year or two apart in age—and not to hire a group of SPs representing both ends of the age range. It does not matter what their *actual* age is as long as they *appear* to be within the age range you are working with. For example, if the training materials for a back pain case require a man of 38 but the age range can be extended from 30 to 50, it is still important to select actors close in age, that is, all who appear to be in their mid- to late 30s or mid- to late 40s, and so on.

Selecting SPs who appear to be the same age makes training and exam administration simpler as well for these reasons:

- All the data in the case relating to the patient's age can be adjusted similarly so that all SPs can be trained with the same information (e.g., years married, ages of children, ages of patient's parents).
- Exam logistics are simpler because only one student instruction sheet (which usually includes the age of the patient) is needed no matter which SP is performing on any given day.

Gender

Decisions about changing the gender of a case must be carefully considered, as must decisions about mixing both male and female SPs playing a given case in the same exam. Although research shows there is little impact of SP and student gender differences on overall test scores (Colliver & Williams, 1993, p. 458), gender differences in performance on specific skills—particularly history-taking and patient/physician interaction—as well as the effect on case content still need to be studied (Petrusa, 2002, pp. 6–7).

Recruit and Train at Least One More Person Than You Anticipate You Will Optimally Need

It is wise to train at least one extra SP as a backup for any program that runs longer than a single event or more than a few days. Many unforeseen circumstances can, and frequently do, arise that keep an SP from participating in an event for which she was trained. The following is an actual situation that illustrates the need for extra coverage, especially for high-stakes examinations. One of the three young women who was recruited and trained for a CPX case that required only two SPs had a gall bladder attack the night before and had to go in for emergency surgery on the first day of the exam. She was out for the duration of the CPX to recover from her operation.

Without a backup person to call on, any situation that keeps an SP from performing could pose serious consequences for a program. It is especially crucial in high-stakes assessments such as an end-of-second-year assessment of the medical students' history taking and physical examination skills, which they are required to pass prior to moving into their third-year required clerkships, or a CPX-type exam, which the students are required to pass in order to graduate from medical school.

Be Sure That all the SPs You Are Recruiting Understand Your Backup Policy

- *Treat all SPs recruited for a given case as equals.* Do not designate the primary SPs you hire as *the performers* while designating the extra SP hired as *the backup*, or as an understudy who will perform only in the event something happens to one of the primary SPs. The SP designated as only a backup will not have as strong a commitment to the training process or to the overall goals of the program as will those who have been hired knowing for sure they are going to perform. In addition, backup SPs who are considered understudies do not have as many opportunities to perform, so their skills in performing the case and accurately filling out the checklist can deteriorate.

- *Plan to train all the SPs together and give each the same number of opportunities to perform, rotating all equally into the assessment events.* Under these guidelines, the SPs feel a similar kind of commitment to the patient case, to the event for which they are being trained, and to the standardized patient program itself. How does this work? If everyone is committed to a given performance schedule, it seems that no one would be free as a backup to fill in if needed. It is important for all SPs to make a commitment to the full timeframe of the examination event even if they will only be working on certain days during that timeframe. Although one SP per case will be performing in any given exam administration, if something happens to the person who was scheduled to perform, there should be at least one other available SP to call on to fill in.

- *Establish a backup policy.* For example, for the days they are not scheduled, require that all SPs remain on call until 7 p.m. the night before the exam. This should be part of the Letter of Agreement the SPs sign before beginning training (see Appendix B1 for a sample of this letter). With the SPs providing backup for each other, the SP coach has the assurance there will be someone available, if needed—and the SPs will have confidence that one of their counterparts will cover for them should the need arise. On the rare occasion that something untoward does come up on the actual day that an SP is scheduled to perform—car trouble, personal illness, illness in the family, and so on—one of the other trained SPs will be able to fill in, even at the last minute.

Look for These Qualities in a New Recruit

- *Acting ability.* The most obvious asset in an SP is her ability to realistically portray the patient. It is also essential to find someone who can take direction, is eager for feedback from the SP coach, and is capable of refocusing her performance so that the patient she is portraying comes to life in the way the SP coach understands the case author's intentions.

- *Self-reflection and keen observation skills.* Even in the midst of a highly emotional performance, the SP must be able to *witness* her interaction with the student as if she were a third person. Based on her observations of the behavior and responses of the student, she must be able to adjust her own behavior and responses as the "patient." This is critical. I have worked with SPs who were superb performers, but who got so involved in their role that they could not accurately remember what had gone on in the encounter, even when they were prompted with questions about the interaction.

  The purpose of a standardized patient performance is to teach or assess the clinical skills of the medical students. It is not solely about the SP's performance ability. If the SP cannot observe the student's behavior and adjust her responses accordingly, the value of the simulated clinical experience is lost. Although we use many techniques of the actor to create a realistic experience, this is not the theater. The SP must use the actor's skill and craft in the service of education and assessment, to enhance the medical student's learning. SP coaches and SPs must always keep this in mind.

- *Ability to accurately recall details of the interaction after the encounter is over.* Observation during the encounter is one thing; being able to recall specific details of the encounter after it is over is another. These are two separate abilities. One can see this in action with an SP who perfectly and appropriately responds to what is going on in the encounter (observation), but, when reflecting on the experience after the encounter is over, cannot accurately remember the details of what transpired. Accurate recall ability in an assessment situation is essential for two reasons:
  - The SP must remember details from the encounter to accurately fill out the case checklist.
  - The SP must remember details of the clinical encounter in order to give effective feedback, in the form of comments from the patient's point of view, about the experience with the medical student.

- *Curiosity about the patient.* The best SPs are genuinely curious about the patient they will be portraying. They want to know who the patient really is and why the patient is responding to the clinical situation in the way the materials suggest. SPs who care about their work in this way will help the SP coach to see where there might be conflicts in the materials or misunderstandings in the checklist.

- *Willingness to work toward standardization of performance with other SPs.* This is not much of an issue when hiring non-actors to perform a case. But the premise under which actors normally operate is different from what we expect of them as standardized patients. In order to get a part, an actor strives to bring a unique, creative interpretation to a character. In other performance arenas, if the actor's interpretation is close enough to what the director is looking for, it is his uniqueness—the quality that makes him stand out from the others auditioned—that gets him the role.

    In our work, however, the actor hired as an SP will be required to incorporate his individual interpretation into the collaborative one that all the SPs performing a given patient role will use. Most actors find this collective approach to a role fascinating and rewarding, but some cannot work this way. Actors hired as SPs must be willing to work cooperatively with the other SPs who are performing the same case so that, together with the SP coach, they can come to a consensus on an interpretation of the patient that ensures the same challenge for all of the medical students being examined no matter which SP any given student might see. Because this is a major change in focus for the actor and a critical mindset for all SPs, actors and non-actors alike should be made explicitly aware of this method of standardization, both during the audition and again *before* training begins.

- *Reliability.* SPs who are valuable assets to any program are those who can be counted on to be on time to every training session and every performance, or who have the courtesy to let the SP coach know as soon as possible when something prevents them from keeping a commitment. We sometimes have a sense of the potential SP's reliability early on in the process. Was the SP late to her audition? Did she call to let you know why she was unable to meet her commitment? Consider eliminating anyone who proves unreliable, no matter what stage of the recruitment–training continuum you are in at the time of the discovery. This is another good reason for training a backup SP. If you have a backup, you will feel more at ease in eliminating an unreliable SP than if you are training only the number of SPs you need.

Recruitment Resources

Recruiting and auditioning on an as-needed basis seem to work best most of the time. Some SP coaches, inclined to preaudition potential SPs before there is a case for them to perform, do so in the hope that it will save time in the future. However, if you audition the potential SP too far in advance of a specific performance, that person might not be available when an appropriate case comes up, or may even need to be re-auditioned, especially if several SPs will be performing the same case.

Even if you audition only when there is a need, encourage anyone who shows interest in your program to send you the same information that you request when you are actively recruiting. Let the person know that you do not conduct auditions until there is a case for which the person might be appropriate, that you have a file on everyone who has shown interest in the program, and that you use that file whenever new recruitment is called for.

Hiring Experienced SPs

Hiring SPs who have already worked in our programs is a common occurrence. A person who can realistically portray a given patient case, who can accurately record student behavior on a checklist, who gives good feedback, who is easy to work with, and/or who is motivated out of a commitment to the educational goals of the program is a person to whom we are naturally inclined to offer additional work. One of the major advantages of employing an experienced SP, whether he is playing a case he has done before or is learning a new one, is that the experienced SP requires less training. If the experienced SP is portraying a case he has performed before, he might only require one or two refresher training sessions. If the experienced SP is learning a new case, he usually requires fewer training sessions and is a quicker study than a new SP who needs to be trained from scratch and needs to be oriented to the general procedures. Another advantage to using experienced SPs is that they are known entities as far as their abilities to maintain consistency in performance and accuracy on the checklists are concerned.

However, if the experienced SP is hired to portray an evaluation case that is similar to a previous one the same SP performed with the students earlier in the curriculum, there is a danger that the students will confuse the two cases if the same SP performs both of them. Here is an example to demonstrate just how vivid these simulated cases can be for students: A student stopped one of our SPs while she was walking across campus to participate in another program. He wanted to know how she was doing and whether her symptoms had resolved. It took the SP aback until she realized the student was referring to a case she had played several months earlier during a teaching demonstration.

This kind of identification of the SP with the patient they are simulating can often carry over from one situation to another. Sometimes this identification of an SP with another case is not a problem. We simply let the students know that they will be seeing SPs they have worked with before, but that they will be portraying different patients. However, the decision making must be more discriminating when casting an assessment case that is similar in nature to one an SP-under-consideration has previously played with the same set of students. For example, it is worth considering not hiring an SP who has played a patient with cardiac symptoms in a teaching case to perform a patient with chest pain in an assessment situation.

Using Referrals From SPs in Your Standardized Patient Pool

Referrals from SPs who are already in your program are the best resource for recruiting. Your SPs know, from experience, the value of the program and what is involved in being a standardized patient. In short, they can be your best recruiting agents. They can also prescreen people because they know and/or have worked with the people they are recommending. They are aware of how easy or how difficult someone might be to work with, whether or not they can be counted on to follow through with training and the performance commitment, whether they can be expected to be on time—all important qualities that are difficult to determine in an audition.

Let all SPs from whom you are asking referrals know that there are multiple actors who are going to be performing the same case for which they are being considered and that there are multiple cases for which you will be casting. Knowing this, the SP will not feel that if he refers another person to you, it might mean he will be in competition with this person and potentially lose the job himself.

Make sure that the SP who makes the referrals knows the qualities you are looking for in the potential new recruits. This might seem unnecessary, but experienced SPs have often commented that they were not aware of all the criteria that were used to hire them initially. Because the SPs are focused on the quality and realism of their performances when doing an audition, they may not be aware of how important other qualities are in the overall scheme (such as the qualities of a new recruit just described).

Encourage the SP making the referrals to contact prospective SPs before you do. Ask the referring SP if she might be willing to

- discuss her experiences as an SP in your program.
- discover whether the person she is referring has an interest in the current project for which you are recruiting.
- determine if the prospective new recruit is available.

Initial contact by the experienced SP can save time by eliminating persons who are not interested or whose schedules conflict with the training or performance requirements. The additional benefit to having the experienced SP contact the new recruits is that the trained SP's description of her personal experience creates an attitude of positive regard toward you and your program before you even talk with the prospective recruits.

Something else to keep in mind is that some SPs will not be willing to give names of potential recruits, as a matter of privacy, until they have contacted the person themselves to determine their interest. If this is the case, ask the SP to give your phone number to the potential recruit. This allows the newcomer an opportunity to think things over before making the decision to contact the program for further information.

If the SP giving you the referrals is unable to make the contact in as timely a fashion as needed by the demands of the program, ask the referring SP's permission to use her name when making your own cold calls to the prospective recruits.

Recruiting Through Outside Agencies

In certain circumstances, it might be necessary to use other methods to recruit SPs for your program. The most obvious situation is when you are setting up a standardized patient program for the first time and do not yet have an SP pool. However, even well-established programs find some of the following methods useful when recruitment-through-referrals does not produce enough new blood to satisfactorily cast a given case.

Outside agencies or organizations (such as a local community theater group, the local chapter of the AARP, etc.) sometimes request that you send a list of requirements that the organization will post for likely candidates to see or that they will print in their next newsletter. Under these conditions, carefully determine what you send. Avoid sending the case itself or detailed descriptions of the case. Too much detail can intimidate a potential recruit. In addition, all SP training materials should be treated as confidential examination materials. You do not want copies of any of your cases in the hands of people who may never participate in your program. At a minimum, the information for posting for recruits needs to include

- a short description of the program.
- a concise description of the demographics and physical character-istics of the patient.
- a line or two about the patient case.
- a deadline for contacting your institution.
- a name and address of the contact person to whom the information should be sent.
- a request for personal information
  - previous experience/resume.
  - why the person is interested in your program.
  - if the potential recruit has any connection with your institution.
  - a photograph (professional head shot or personal snapshot).

Recruiting Using Newspapers/Newsletters

The greatest advantage to this form of recruitment is the potential for identifying interested people with whom you would otherwise not come in contact. There are two types of newspaper exposure for SP recruiting:

(a) ads taken out by the standardized patient program for specific needs and
(b) articles done on your SP program or on one of your standardized patients by a journalist.

The more focused the audience of a newspaper or newsletter, the better the chance you have of getting responses from the kind of people you are seeking. For example, if you need older men for a geriatric case, contacting the local senior citizen center and putting information into their newsletter assures you that those who respond will be in the right age group. The larger the circulation of the newspaper, the more likely it is that the responses you receive will be eclectic. You will probably get a large volume of phone calls that run the gamut from the outright bizarre to the merely curious to those who have true potential. If you are in a large metropolitan area, you can avoid this barrage of telephone calls by requesting that correspondence be sent to a post office box.

With either type of newspaper promotion, be sure to request that interested parties send

- a photograph.
- a resume of acting or other related experiences (such as teaching, police undercover work, etc.).

- a letter of interest explaining
  - how they found out about the program.
  - why they are interested in doing simulated patient work.
  - a little bit about themselves (leave this part of the request open-ended to see what the potential SP is inclined to share with you).

The replies you receive will provide you with enough information to decide which individuals to contact.

Recruiting From Health-Related Support Groups

Other valuable places for finding potential recruits include support groups or organizations whose membership focuses on a specific health issue such as arthritis, diabetes, hypertension control, and so on. However, among these groups are certain categories of persons who require special consideration in regard to SP work:

- *Persons with mental disorders.* Certain of these patients can work in teaching situations when one is looking for real patients to work with the students. However, avoid hiring anyone as a standardized patient who cannot respond appropriately based on the case framework and give constructive feedback to the students. On the other hand, caregivers of persons with mental disorders often make excellent standardized patients for both teaching and assessment purposes because they have lived with the effects of the illness on a daily basis. They frequently bring nuances to their performances that others, not in their situation, would not even know to include. Look for them in caregiver support groups of the specific disorder you are trying to cast, such as Alzheimer's disease support groups for dementia.

- *The physically challenged.* Physically challenged patients often have physical characteristics and findings that are impossible to simulate, such as swollen joints, heart murmurs, enlarged livers, atrophied muscles, diminished pulses, and so on. However, persons who are physically challenged pose a different kind of decision making at the time of recruitment for standardized patient assessment cases. It is important to think about how the person's real deficits might affect his ability to perform under all the circumstances of the case's use. Can the person separate himself enough from his own story to be able to take on the characteristics of the standardized patient case? Additional considerations depend on the specific physical deficit and the stamina of the person who has the deficit. Will the requirements of the case performance be too much for the patient to endure? For example, can the real patient endure eight encounters with eight different students in a 3- or 4-hour period?

- *The terminally ill.* Carefully interview anyone who has a terminal illness before hiring them to portray a case with similar characteristics. For example, some patients with renal failure are willing to share their experiences of their illness, and by doing so know that they are providing a service to the medical community. But hiring persons who are on dialysis to talk about their own illness in a learning environment versus hiring the same person to portray a standardized patient for a clinical skills assessment can be very different. In talking about their own illnesses in a teaching setting, persons with a terminal illness often are given permission to maneuver around issues that are too painful for them to discuss, whereas these same issues might be the very ones they would be required to deal with in a standardized patient assessment case.

  Some terminally ill persons with AIDS, cancer, COPD (chronic obstructive lung disease), or another disease, who believe they have resolved their issues around death, may discover in the process of learning and performing the standardized patient case with the students, that their fears are stirred anew. This can be difficult for everyone involved, but especially for the person with the terminal illness.

  It is not only terminally ill patients for whom these kinds of issues arise. More often than one might expect, SPs find themselves hired for roles that are very close to home, for example:

> A new standardized patient was hired to portray a young woman who has a duodenal ulcer. In the patient case, the young woman fears that she has been misdiagnosed and that she really has stomach cancer as her mother who died a year earlier had. The SP learned the case with ease and performed it realistically in training, but the second day of the exam, she became withdrawn and uncommunicative when she was not performing the case. Even though her portrayal and checklists were of high quality, it was clear that something was not right. As it turned out, her father had died of stomach cancer the year before, and he had died in the very hospital in which we were doing the exam. When I asked her why she hadn't told us this, she said that she thought doing the case would help her get over her grieving, but she actually realized that performing the case in the same hospital in which he had died was just too much for her.

Ever since that experience, we have asked potential SPs—who are going to perform a patient who either has a terminal illness or who fears her symptoms might mean "something serious is going on"—if there is anything in the case that relates to anything they have experienced before. If there is something else, we explore why the SP wants to perform the case and try to determine what would be in the best interest of the SP and the program. The answer is not to reject all SPs whose lives have similar issues as the case. Some SPs will do an excellent job with the case *because* of their life experiences with terminal illness.

It all depends on the specifics of the situation. However we look at it, knowing about issues in the case that relate to the SP's life is important information for us because these connections can help us to assist the SP in giving an authentic performance. I suspect that the young woman in the previous example might have been able to play the same case a few years later using her experience with her father as the source to create a truly authentic performance without the personal emotional upset. In her situation, the timing was just not right. It was too soon—or, then again, it might never have been right.

Recruiting From Volunteer Organizations

You can recruit from such organizations, especially those related to health care or to the specifics of the patient case. Take this example: The patient case requires finding a middle-age woman who works as a docent for the local zoo and is coming to see the doctor because of a chronic cough. Talk to the docents at the local zoo!

Recruiting From Schools of the Performing Arts

The most obvious group to look for SPs is among actors. Besides their inherent performance abilities, actors who are not making a living exclusively as performers have other jobs that give them the flexibility to attend auditions and participate in performances.

Recruiting From Other Professions With Flexible Schedules

Professions with flexible time schedules can be fertile ground for finding people who would be competent SPs: firemen, policemen, stay-at-home parents, active senior citizens, parent/teacher associations (PTAs), elementary/high school teachers (especially during the summer break), and college faculty.

Teachers, as a group, are generally very effective SPs. Good teachers are natural actors. They have to be in order to be effective communicators. Teachers also know better than most how to give feedback because it is part of their responsibility as teachers. Coaching SPs to give effective feedback is one of the more challenging aspects of the training process, so being able to work with teachers who already understand how to provide feedback makes this part of the job that much easier.

Recruitment Procedures

Start Recruitment 6 to 8 Weeks Prior to SP Training

If the examination consists of eight or more cases, you need at least 6 to 8 weeks to find the number of people necessary. Events of the magnitude of a CPX usually require going beyond the experienced pool of SPs to find the necessary complement of performers. Even if the exam remains exactly the same from one year to the next, the availability of the SPs who previously portrayed the cases will probably have changed.

Give yourself the time you think you need in order to do an adequate job of recruitment, even if all were to go well—then add a couple of weeks for the inevitable. It is always a good idea to leave more time to recruit than you think it will take. Otherwise you risk being caught by a training deadline and thus forced to select some people who in other circumstances you would not have. Under this kind of pressure, it is easy to become good at rationalizing why a person might be just fine: "Maybe I had a bad day during the audition," "Maybe his inability to adequately fill out the checklist will improve," "Maybe her initial discomfort about having a physical exam won't affect her performance," or "Maybe that teenager's look of defiance doesn't mean he'll be difficult to work with." In short, you get caught making "maybe" decisions.

Many of us have found ourselves in this unpleasant position. But some years ago, after trying countless times to work with people whom I had chosen against my better judgment, I gave up casting patients out of the give-them-the-benefit-of-the-doubt method and began to trust my intuition. It was not easy to do, especially when I could not articulate my misgivings about certain candidates. Making decisions based on intuition is often difficult. We are always second guessing ourselves, especially when we are facing a deadline. It took years of living with bad decisions in recruiting to finally give myself permission to pay attention to my instincts.

To Save Time, Recruit on the Telephone

When interviewing a potential candidate, do the following:

- *Explain the program and the specific goals of the case for which you are recruiting.*

- *Ask explicitly if the person is interested in the project.* Do this early in the phone call. It might save you from giving the rest of your prepared speech to someone who is not really interested and is only being polite.

- *Encourage the candidate to send in a picture and resume along with a note stating why he thinks he might like to participate in the program.*

- *Engage the candidate in conversation so that you can discover something about him.* Ask how he found out about the program. Explore what interests him about the job or what makes him feel he would like to participate.

- *Find out the candidate's attitude toward the medical profession, especially any negative experiences the person might have had.* If you ask about this directly, the candidate might surmise that you are looking for a positive answer and adapt her response to fit what she thinks you want to hear. However, if you trust that at some point in your conversation the candidate will bring up a personal experience with a physician or other health care professional, you can wait until that moment and then invite her to tell you more about her experiences. If the subject does not come up naturally, you can simply ask the potential SP something neutral such as, "What kind of experiences have you had with the medical profession?" It is better not to hire someone who has a quarrel with an individual physician or negative feelings toward the medical profession, because there is a good possibility that this kind of person will end up transferring that anger and expressing it in the SP work they do for your program. Having said this, I suggest that before making up your mind to eliminate a candidate, carefully listen to the description of the negative experience with an ear to sensing whether the person has worked through her feelings and will be able to constructively use that experience in shaping her work on the patient case and in giving feedback to the students.

- *Determine the candidate's availability for both training and performance.* Simply ask the candidate whether his schedule is flexible enough to accommodate the specific inclusive dates you have identified for both training and administration of the examination.

- *Discuss the physical examination requirement.* Even if the candidate will be auditioning for a case that only involves history taking, for future reference determine how the person feels about:
  - wearing a patient gown.
  - having a physical examination of the type required by all cases for which the candidate is being considered. If the physical examination requires exposure of intimate parts of the body (for example, a cardiac exam required on a woman), find out for sure before auditioning the candidate that she understands the kinds of physical exposure necessary during an exam. Be sure that the candidate knows and agrees to have medical students perform all physical maneuvers necessary to accomplish a thorough physical examination, even if those maneuvers are not explicitly mentioned in the training materials or the checklist.

- *Provide limited case information before the audition.* Many candidates will ask you for some details of the case so that they can do some preparation before coming to the audition. To this reasonable request, you may offer them the following information over the telephone:
  - the medical problem of the case you anticipate asking the candidate to audition for, such as back pain, diabetes, or headache.
  - a description of the patient's emotional tone and attitude toward the clinic visit.
  - a bit of personal background on the patient (backstory).
  With this information, the candidates can do some preliminary work before the audition. Based on what you share with them, some may even come dressed in what they think the patient might wear. This kind of preparation by candidates is instructive. It shows you how seriously they view the audition and gives you a sense of their potential value as a standardized patient.

- *Let all the candidates know, prior to the audition, that everyone will do a cold reading (an interview from material given to them on the spot) from a synopsis of the case that they will get during orientation at the audition.* The synopsis will include more detailed patient information than you have shared with them verbally during the telephone recruitment (see Appendix A10).

- *Inform the recruits about video recording.* Let the candidates know that all practice encounters during training and the Practice Exam will be video recorded as will all clinical encounters with the medical students during the actual CPX. Letting the candidates know about video recording is purely informational at this point, but you want to find out now if they are comfortable with this requirement and if not, eliminate them from your list of candidates.

- *Check all the critical demographics of the case.* Make sure the candidate is the appropriate age, weight, and ethnicity. Find out if the candidate has any medical problems, including physical illnesses, prior surgeries, scars, and the like that might confound the case.

- *Find out if the candidate knows, or has a relationship with, any of the students in your medical school.* Decide whether or not such a relationship might compromise your program.

- *Discuss payment schedule.* Let the candidate know what compensation he will receive for the training and for each administration of the exam. Determine whether or not the amount of payment is agreeable to the candidate. Should he seem unhappy with what the pay will be, consider not auditioning him.

  You might mention your hourly rate on the telephone. But to avoid problems of misinterpretation once the candidate is hired, it is prudent to also name a lump sum that the SP will receive for each training session and each exam administration performance. Here is an example of why thinking about and explaining payment in this way is important.

  Let's say you want the SPs to perform for $3\frac{1}{2}$ hours each time they work in the clinical exam. However, you want them to show up $\frac{1}{2}$ hour before the exam to get ready for their performances and to stay 15 minutes after the exam to debrief with you. Therefore, you intend to pay them for $4\frac{1}{4}$ hours of participation. But if you do not give them a lump sum figure, some SPs will assume you are paying them for every minute they are present, and some will even assume you are paying them for the time it takes them to drive to and from your exam center!

  A good way to assure that the candidates you finally select for a given program understand exactly what they will be getting paid is to put this information in writing in the form of a letter of agreement (see Appendix B1). It makes the communication clear, and you have something in writing to refer to if any misunderstandings arise.

- *Schedule the candidate for an audition.* If the candidate seems appropriate, schedule a time for her to come in and audition. If you are unsure or need more time to make a decision about whether or not the candidate is right for SP work, let her know you will be calling her back to schedule an audition after reviewing her information with your team (e.g., assistant coach, CPX advisory committee, faculty consultant).

One final reminder: Recruitment may continue throughout the auditioning process. Do not be surprised if you are still recruiting until the first day of training, even if that is not how you planned it. As part of recruitment, ask every person who auditions if they know anyone else who might be right for any of the cases you have yet to cast.

AUDITIONING

The term audition is defined as "a trial performance, as by an actor, to demonstrate suitability or skill" (*American Heritage Dictionary*, 1997, p. 90). Besides determining which candidates have the capability of performing the case, SP coaches have additional reasons for auditioning. We also need to determine whether the candidate can carry out the other responsibilities of a standardized patient, which are to accurately fill out a checklist and give appropriate verbal or written feedback. That is why it is so important to go through the necessary effort to set up an audition. One casting director put it this way: We go through auditions "because no one has ever devised a better way to cast. If you think of one, let us know.... It's not a surefire method, of course, how could anything so subjective be certain?... but it's the only way we've got" (Shurtleff, 1978, p. 22).

The best way to determine the level of each candidate's skills is by a mini-performance in all three areas: (a) portrayal capability, (b) accuracy, and (c) giving feedback. Auditioning can be an insightful and rewarding experience that everyone enjoys, or it can be chaotic and only marginally beneficial, frustrating all the participants. What makes the difference is organization and attitude—the way the audition is coordinated and the mindset of the auditioning staff toward the candidates. This is the heart of the auditioning process.

Auditioning Principles

Because auditioning is essential for finding and getting the best SP candidates, I offer the following guidelines.

When to Audition

Auditioning can start as soon as there are enough candidates to do so. If the case is straightforward, four is a practical number to audition at any one time. If the case has simulated physical findings that need to be auditioned or more complex performance requirements, consider scheduling three candidates for a single auditioning session to give yourself more time with each candidate.

Whenever Practical, Schedule Only Candidates Who Seem Right for a Specific Case

Although it is not always logistically possible to do this, it makes orientation and selection easier if you can audition multiple candidates who seem right for the same case. It allows you to compare performances in the immediacy of a single auditioning session, rather than have to review video recordings or recall performances from scattered sessions over the course of several days.

Complete Auditioning at Least 1 Week Before Training Is Scheduled to Begin

During the week or so before training starts, you should make the final selection of SPs and call those who have been chosen in order to confirm the schedule for the first training session.

Set Up the Auditioning Environment for Both Efficiency and Comfort

Because the purpose of an audition is to find the most capable candidates for each of the patient cases, create a well-organized, but friendly, environment that will allow the candidates to perform at their optimum so that you can get a sense of the true expertise of each person you audition. This means that your staff must understand how important it is to be helpful and supportive in their interactions with the candidates. Harold Prince, a well-known theater producer–director, says that what he is looking for in his assistant is "someone who loves actors, someone who understands the problem of actors looking for work.... Someone who roots for the actor, wants every actor to get that job" (Hunt, 1977, p. 172).

One can easily become overwhelmed by the logistical demands and forget that the bottom line is finding the most suitable people to perform the cases. As you are setting up the process, or when you are feeling overloaded, it helps to ask yourself, "Is this procedure going to elicit the best performance each candidate is capable of?"

Be Aware of What the Candidates Usually Experience at an Audition

According to Gordon Hunt (1977), who was casting director for the Mark Taper Forum in Los Angeles when he wrote a book for actors called *How to Audition*, the anticipation a candidate experiences is something like this:

You are sitting on a hard metal chair in some hallway or waiting room. Your palms sweat. Your heartbeat has increased by a third. Pangs of fear dit-dat across your chest, down to your stomach and back up to the chest again. Your mouth is dry. Your hands shake, and when you stand, your knees tremble. Breath is short. You sweat. Your mind clouds over. For all you know or care, your life could end at that moment, and no one, especially you, would mind too much. As a matter of fact, death might be a blessed relief.

The above is not from a [prisoner of war] about to undergo interrogation or a patient waiting for a life or death diagnosis or a convict about to be sentenced for a capital crime. It's you... to a greater or lesser degree... it is you... about to go through that agonizing life-or-death process known as the audition. (p. 1)

Hunt has captured the universal experience of a person going through an audition. It applies as much to those auditioning for a standardized patient role as it does to anyone else, skilled actor or not, who has ever auditioned for a part in anything, whether it be a high school play, the local community theater, Broadway, television, or a Hollywood film. Besides the anxiety that everyone who goes through the auditioning process has, it is "potentially a humiliating experience" (Hunt, p. 172). No matter how supportive the environment is, what always looms in the background for the candidate is possible rejection.

Always Audition Before Casting a New Case

Even if we are considering casting people we have worked with before, it is still worth having them audition for a new patient case. It is hard to know even how an experienced SP will do on another type of case, especially if the new case requires a different kind of personality or emotional performance from what the SP has done before.

Try to Keep an Open Mind

Type-casting is unfair to both the candidates and to ourselves. Sometimes certain SPs are eliminated from consideration because we start to think of them only for the types of patient cases they have already performed. In fact, we might fail to cast an excellent internal candidate because of a preconception we have about her. If this happens too often, there is a good chance the candidate might start to get stale in her performances because she has never been given an opportunity to stretch herself and use her range of skills.

During auditions, I have often been surprised at the extent of some SPs' capabilities. This is because I had assumed I knew what they were capable of, simply because I had been working with them for some time. The surprise came, not because the SPs were suddenly better than they had ever been, but because I had not yet given them an opportunity to demonstrate the scope of their talent in the patient cases they had been performing.

Do not be fooled by how the candidate *looks*. A person might look exactly the way we imagined the patient to look but turn out to be absolutely wrong for the case. If we hold preconceived notions about those who are auditioning, our work with them will not have the openness that allows us to see other qualities that are actually there.

Audition No More Than Four Candidates at Any One Time

Respect for the candidates' time (remember, they are not being paid to audition) and efficiency for those holding the auditions are two criteria to use when deciding how many candidates to audition at any given session. If too many candidates are called in at the same time, some of them will have to wait an unreasonable amount of time before they get to audition.

Record Every Audition on Video

It is important to video record every audition for several reasons:

- The videos are a record of the auditions, which can be reviewed by you and your selection committee when making final decisions.
- It is a sign of your seriousness about the auditioning process, and the candidates know you will have documentation of their performances to refer to, if necessary, rather than rely on memory alone.

At the Audition Never Give the Candidates an Indication Whether or Not They Have Been Chosen

Harold Prince makes a keen observation about how easily we can fall into "misleading" the candidates after the audition is over:

> The actor must not leave ... thinking he got the job because you were so nice to him—because you did the equivalent of applauding him no matter what you thought of him. ... That's as dishonest and, in a funny way, as damaging as treating him badly. So you are treading a thin line. (Hunt, 1977, p. 173)

This observation is key: It is important to be both accommodating and truthful. It might seem that the simplest way to handle the auditions would be to praise everybody because it provides a nice, polite way to say goodbye to the candidate. However, it is unfair to give the candidates an idea that they might be cast for a case when, in truth, even you cannot know until all the auditions are over whether a given candidate will be selected or not. A simple, straightforward "thank you," along with information on when the candidate can expect to hear the results of the audition, is respectful and all that is required.

Even if you are enthusiastic about a potential SP who auditioned well, resist the temptation to cast on the spot. The selection process should happen after you have auditioned all potential candidates for several reasons:

- More frequently than one might imagine, in subsequent auditions someone else embodies the patient better than the person you were inclined to cast earlier.
- The notion of standardization changes as we audition the pool of candidates; for example, we decide on a particular body type because several of the other candidates have the same build, or we choose candidates at the upper end of the patient's age range rather than at the lower end.

Everybody Needs Time to Reflect

It is a good idea to give the candidates time to reflect on the case, what you have told them about the requirements of the clinical examination, the pay, and the commitment in terms of training and performances. Sometimes a candidate who would have accepted the role in the excitement of the audition will later decide not to participate for various personal reasons.

Not hiring in the excitement of an excellent audition is a hard rule to follow, but virtually every time I have cast out of the enthusiasm of the moment, I have regretted it. To remind myself, I keep a sheet of paper in my audition folder that says NOT NOW!

Auditioning Logistics

The time to allot for an auditioning session is $1\frac{1}{2}$ to 2 hours. The candidates themselves should not be kept for more than 1 hour. If you plan to audition any of the candidates for multiple cases, factor in extra time for them. In fact, if you need more time for the auditions for any reason, schedule three candidates per session rather than four.

Suggested Schedule

The following schedule is an example of how to allot time to the various activities for an uncomplicated, straightforward, one-candidate-per-single-case auditioning session:

10 minutes: SP coach orients group of candidates, having them fill out a Standardized Patient Profile Form (see sample in Appendix B2).

10 minutes: Candidates review the case summary and abridged checklist—documents that have been prepared specifically for the audition from the case materials (see samples in Appendixes A10 and A11)—and ask questions.

40 minutes: Auditions—10 minutes per individual.

20 minutes: SP coach discusses audition with assistant. Production notes are recorded on the candidate's profile form (either after each candidate leaves the audition or at the end of the session)—5 minutes per candidate.

10 minutes: Time that can be spread out and used with any candidate who might need more direction during an individual audition.

1½ hours: Total time spent in the auditioning session. (Give yourself 30–45 minutes between auditioning sessions to review your notes and prepare for the next session.)

Physical Layout

Two rooms should be set aside for the auditioning process. One should be large enough for all the candidates and staff to gather for orientation. This area (a small conference room works well) can also be the place where the candidates fill out paperwork, have Polaroid and/or digital photographs taken, and await their turn to audition. The other room is the actual auditioning area. It need only be large enough for

- three people (the candidate, the SP coach, and the assistant).
- a video camera.
- an examination table or a gurney (for auditioning the more complicated physical examination simulations).

Personnel

If possible, I advise having two other people to help you carry out the tasks of each auditioning session: an assistant to work with you during the auditions themselves and a manager to handle all of the administrative details, including the comings and goings of the candidates. These would be their responsibilities:

1. The SP coach. The SP coach might do general orientation of the candidates but should participate in the auditioning of each candidate, if possible.
2. The assistant/observer. This person will
   - create an environment of safety, "protecting" the candidates by being a witness. This is particularly important if physical exam simulations are required in the audition.
   - label and prepare the videos/DVDs, or program the digital video software for use during the auditions. Dedicate a video/DVD to each case with a list of the candidates in the order they appear. If you do not have digital video files, this procedure will make it easier to find candidates, compare their performances, or verify your casting decisions (so that you do not have to rely on your memory or notes) during the selection process after the auditions are complete.
   - set up equipment and record video for each candidate.
   - fill out a copy of the case checklist while the SP coach is doing the audition interview with the candidate. (Having the assistant fill out the checklist frees the coach to focus on the candidate's performance and other aspects of the audition itself.) The assistant's checklist will be used by the coach to compare responses with the checklist that the candidate will fill out after the interview (see Appendix A11, Audition Abridged Checklist).
   - review impressions of the candidate's abilities with the coach and take performance notes on the SP Profile Form (some coaches prefer to do this task themselves) after each audition and/or at the end of the auditioning session (see Appendix B2).
3. The manager. Besides welcoming the candidates, the manager will
   - take Polaroid and/or digital photographs of each of the candidates. Printed photos are beneficial to have during the auditioning process to help you remember what the candidate looked like. Digital images are useful because they can be scanned into the demographic information files in your standardized patient computer database.
   - make sure the candidates fill out the SP Profile Form and a video slate. If you do not have a digital video marking system, the simplest way to keep track of each person recorded on video is to create a visual slate by having each candidate print his name in block letters with a marking pen on an $8\frac{1}{2} \times 11$ piece of paper.

Before the audition begins, the assistant starts the video camera and asks the candidate to say his name while holding the slate up to the camera in front of himself. Because the visual slate can be easily seen in the fast forward mode on video playback, it makes it easy to find specific auditions on the video or DVD should you need to review several candidates' performances.

- attach the video slate and the Polaroid photo to the Profile Form for the candidate to take into the audition.
- provide refreshments, put the candidates at their ease, and answer questions while they are waiting for their turn to audition. During this process, without the coach present, the manager can get a sense of the potential SPs when they are not performing, a sense of them as individuals, and of how easy or how difficult it might be to work with them.
- say good-bye to the candidates and confirm when they can expect to hear whether or not they have been selected.

Neither the assistant nor the manager need be regular members of the SP training program. The main criteria to look for when bringing support personnel on board to facilitate auditioning are enthusiasm for the program, understanding of the goals of the auditions, and good people skills so that their presence helps to put the candidates in the frame of mind to do their best work.

Selection Committee

The purpose of forming this committee is to provide the SP coach with trusted, informed colleagues whose advice can be sought when there are difficult decisions to make regarding specific candidates. This committee might simply consist of you and another coach, but it could include other consultants such as the case author or one of the clinicians on the CPX advisory committee. (For more details on selection of candidates, see the corresponding section which follows.)

Auditioning Materials

The following are important materials to have available when auditioning.

The SP Profile Form

The data on this form include the basic information that you will keep on file for each standardized patient in your program. You can keep this information in a casting book (see the next section), but it is also important to transfer this information into a computer database, which will allow you to update information easily and keep track of the cases each SP has performed. Once the information (in the *Auditioned For* section of the profile form) is in the database, you can retrieve the names of all the SPs who have performed a given case and easily determine how recently each has portrayed the case and whether a refresher session or retraining is in order.

The last section on the SP Profile Form is for written comments about the candidate. It is in this section that the coach or the assistant will take performance notes based on your discussions of the candidates after the auditions. These comments will jog your memory when it comes time to make the final selection decisions.

Regardless of whether the candidates have brought photos of themselves, the manager should take a close-up head shot of all candidates by Polaroid and/or digital camera while they are waiting for their audition. These photographs are often better representations of the physical appearance of the candidates than the professional photographs they bring in. Keep the printed photos attached to the candidates' profile form for use when making your final selections.

Casting Aids

Here are a couple of ideas you might find helpful in keeping track of the candidates you are considering throughout the casting process.

- *Photo mural.* As you audition, keep an ongoing wall display of the top candidates' photographs. Line up the photos underneath the name of the case for which you are considering casting the candidate. This photo mural becomes an ongoing selection board, which is a quick visual reminder of who is being considered to play which cases. This visual display—which will ultimately reflect the final SPs chosen to portray all the cases—is even helpful to have up throughout training, especially if you have multiple projects going on.

- *Casting book.* Following the selection of the candidates, place the completed Profile Form with the Polaroid photograph, along with the head shot and resume of each candidate, in a casting book (three-ring binders work well). You can refer to these photographs and the notes you took on the Profile Form to refresh your memory about the individuals you have auditioned who might be right for future patient cases. You might also want to file photographs of persons who have shown an interest in the SP program, even though you might not yet have had an opportunity to audition them for a suitable case. Having an electronic version of your casting book in the form of a standardized patient computer database (which includes digital images and the information from the Profile Form) is equally useful. Both the electronic and hard copy versions of the information complement each other well.

Case Summaries

The candidates cannot audition without information about the patient. It appears, at first glance, that the easiest way to handle this need would be to give the candidates the case training materials. However, it is unwise to give out the full set of the training materials before or during the audition for two reasons:

- The training materials are a strategic resource in the medical education program, especially if they are part of a clinical skills examination; therefore, these case documents must be handled as secure materials and should not be given to anyone who has not been contracted to perform a given case.
- Because the training materials should not be released to anyone who is not actively studying a case for which they have been selected, one option for the tryouts would be to give the training materials to the candidate at the time of the audition. However, this can be overwhelming because there is generally too much information to assimilate in the time allotted before the candidate is called into the audition.

What I recommend instead is to prepare a case summary for the audition (see Appendix A10). What you include in the case summary depends largely on the case. The summary can be as short as a couple of paragraphs but no more than two or three pages and is given to the candidate during the audition orientation. The case summary might include the following information, which can be taken from the training materials:

- the patient's primary reason for the clinic visit and how the patient responds to the student's opening inquiry, "What brings you to the clinic today?"
- some of the more pertinent historical facts of the present illness.
- information about the patient's affect and emotional tone during the visit.
- some personal background about the patient (so that the candidate understands the context within which the clinic visit is being made).

An Abridged Version of the Checklist

Along with the case summary, the candidates should get a condensed version of the history and physical exam sections of the case checklist to study just before their audition (see Appendix A11). What you need to know in an audition about the candidate's ability to use a checklist can be determined from their completion of the abbreviated history portion of the checklist because it has information about the patient that must be handled in a specific manner during the clinical encounter with the medical student. Auditioning the case using this abbreviated checklist (and having the candidate fill out the history section after the interview) will help you determine whether or not the candidate

- has a tendency to volunteer checklist information to the student.
- can accurately observe and recall the interviewer's behavior after the encounter is over.
- has a global understanding and rationale for how she answered each checklist item.

If you are auditioning anyone new to standardized patient work, always encourage questions from them about the physical exam items so any issues that might have arisen in their review of the materials can be dealt with during the audition. If the case has physical findings that must be simulated, it is imperative to audition all the candidates to determine whether or not they can actually produce the findings that are needed. Otherwise there is generally no need to audition the physical exam or have the candidates fill out the physical exam portion of the checklist. (There is more on this subject in what follows.)

Auditioning Orientation for the Candidates

Activities Before and During Orientation

As the candidates arrive, collect their photographs and resumes. Have them fill out the SP Profile Form and a video slate. Even though you have probably asked all of the questions on this form during recruitment, it is wise to have your assistant or manager look over the profile forms the candidates have just completed to determine if there is any information that would be useful for you to know before starting the auditions. It is particularly important to look at the question on scars or other physical findings. When a candidate answers this question over the telephone, he might not think to mention a chronic condition he has been living with since his youth or a scar he has from surgery that was performed years ago, but when he comes to the audition and is asked to fill out the form, there it is! For example:

> Once during recruitment an older man indicated that the only physical findings he had were related to his lower back problems (which we came to find out later was what he was most concerned about at the time he was asked this question on the telephone). However, when he filled out the physical findings section of the demographic form at the audition, he indicated that he had an appendectomy scar. Because we were planning to audition this candidate for an abdominal pain case that required a physical examination, we could no longer consider him to portray this patient because his appendectomy scar would have confounded the case.

Consequently, it is important to have this information before you hand out the various case scenarios. In a situation like the one just described, there are several options: (a) You can decide to go ahead and audition the candidate in the original case, just to get an idea of his abilities for future projects; (b) if you have another case whose demographics the candidate fits, you can switch gears and audition him for that one; or (c) you can thank the candidate and tell him you will call when you have another case that might be suitable for him.

Information to Cover During Orientation

Some of the material to cover during the opening of orientation will be information you have already discussed with the candidates during the recruitment process. This might seem a duplication of effort. However, it is important to repeat the critical information because occasionally the candidates do not register what you have said over the phone or, as we have just seen, they have forgotten to tell you something crucial that will affect their suitability to perform a case. Briefly explain the following:

- *The case.* How the case for which they are auditioning fits into the overall clinical teaching or assessment protocols of the medical school curriculum.

- *The video recording.* Let the candidates know that video recording is standard procedure during auditioning, throughout training, and is also part of the protocol during the examination. Mention that the video recordings will be used by a committee that has been specifically set up to aid in the selection process.

- *The physical examination.* Explain that most cases require the medical students to perform a physical examination on the patient (SP) and that some cases require the SPs to simulate physical findings (give examples), which means it will be necessary for the SPs portraying those cases to wear a gown and have a physical examination done on them while they are being recorded on video. Be sure to ask again if anyone has a problem with this. More than once, we have had candidates tell us that they understood that some cases would require a physical exam, but they did not realize that they would have to wear a patient gown.

- *Availability.* Double check the candidates' availability for the dates of training and performances. On occasion, a candidate might reveal in orientation that they will be unavailable for certain dates that you had already confirmed with them. Depending on the seriousness of the scheduling conflicts, you will have to decide whether you want to audition the candidate anyway or wait to audition him later when his schedule is more compatible with your training program and performance schedules.

- *Case summaries and checklists.* Hand out case summaries and abbreviated checklists to the candidates. Discuss the information on the checklist and how it relates to the facts of the case. Emphasize that they are not to volunteer anything on the checklist and that they are only to give checklist information if the interviewer specifically asks for it. Address the importance of the checklist in assessing the clinical competence of the students.

- *Accuracy requirement.* Let the candidates know that their ability to accurately complete the checklist—based on what happened in the clinical encounter—is as important as their ability to perform the case. Let them know that, as part of the audition, they will be filling out an abridged version of the checklist (see Appendix A11) immediately after their interview and will be going over it with the SP coach before they leave the audition.

- *Background on SPs in medical education.* Give copies of articles about standardized patients to the candidates to read while they are waiting for their turn to audition. Try to find articles that will give them a feel for the type of work they will be doing as standardized patients. Articles from your own local newspaper are best, but if none are available, there are many published articles that describe the contribution that standardized patients are making to the education of the next generation of physicians. (Look for articles in major newspapers such as *The New York Times*, *The Chicago Tribune*, *The Los Angeles Times*, or from any large city near you that has a medical school with an SP program.)

- *The audition.* Briefly discuss the audition protocol as described in the following section.

The Audition

During the audition, you will be looking to hire candidates who have similar physical characteristics and who give the most realistic portrayal of the patients. But it is equally important to discover

- how well the candidates take direction.
- how perceptive they are in their understanding of the patient.
- how capable they are of not volunteering information on the checklist.
- how accurate they are in filling out the checklist.
- how thoughtful they are in their responses to missed items on the checklist.
- how capable they are of producing the simulated aspects of the physical findings.
- how they interact with you and your assistant.

The Auditioning Schedule

The audition interview of each candidate should take no more than 2 to 3 minutes. The rest of the 10 minutes allotted to the audition can be used for coaching, checklist recording and discussion, conversation, and physical examination simulation, if necessary.

The Auditioning Protocol

The SP coaches know the cases best and the qualities they are looking for in the candidates, so it is ideal to have them involved by doing the following:

- *Invite each candidate one by one into the audition room.* Your assistant can take the SP Profile Form, photograph, and resume from the candidate while you do the welcoming.
- *Start the audition with a brief conversation.* The conversation should be on a topic that has nothing to do with the case the person is trying out for. Besides helping to put the person at ease so that they can perform at their best, you can achieve other goals through this dialogue, one of the most important of which is to get a feel for the kind of person the candidate is and whether or not you would like to work with the person. This initial conversation might include some of the same screening questions you asked over the telephone during recruitment:
  – how the prospective SP found out about the program.
  – the kinds of experiences he has had with doctors.
  – if he works with or knows anyone at your medical school.

Ask these questions informally so that the SP can answer without trying to anticipate what you are looking for. If the candidate has an affiliation with any of the students, it could put him in a compromising situation. SPs naturally want to share information about what they are doing as standardized patients. This is not so risky if the SP is working on a teaching case, but it could jeopardize the clinical skills examination if the SP were to share any information on an assessment case. Therefore, to be safe, and not put the candidate in an awkward situation, do not hire anyone who has an affiliation with a current medical student.

If the prospective SP answers any of the aforementioned topics in a way that makes you uncomfortable, do not let the candidate know your reactions. It is better to go through with the audition, get a sense of the candidate's capabilities, and make a decision about this other information later on.

- *Set the scene for the audition.* Ask the prospective SP if she has any questions about the case. Review the key features of the audition:
  - a brief interview (with the candidate in the role of the patient; you in the role of the medical student). Candidates are usually worried about getting all the facts correct. Let them know that you are not as concerned about the facts as about the realism of their portrayal. There will be time to work on the facts during training.
  - completion of an abbreviated checklist.
  - review of the checklist with the candidate.

- *Ask the candidate to let your assistant know when she is ready to begin the audition.* Give the prospective SP control of the start of the audition. Remember if you are not recording digital video, the candidate will need to mark the start of her audition by saying her real name to the camera while holding the video slate chest high. Some candidates may then want a moment to get into character; others will be ready to begin immediately.

- *Do not try to do a perfect interview with the candidates.* Be sure to ask some open-ended questions and to leave out some items on the checklist. You want to give them an opportunity to interact with you and use information about the patient without volunteering checklist items. At the same time, you want to challenge the SP to remember what actually happened in the encounter and not just to go down the checklist and mark "yes" on every item.

- *If you are unsure about any of the candidates during the audition, talk with them, coach them, then give them another chance to perform.* Do not let a candidate who has potential leave because she did not give you, on the spot, the performance you were looking for. If you are uncertain about someone's interpretation, take the time during their audition to talk with them about what you have observed. If something the potential SP is doing is completely off the mark, you can even stop the interview midstream and discuss your concerns. However, be careful not to stop the interview too early in the process. You want to give the candidates enough time to get beyond audition anxiety and move into their sense of the patient and their capability with the role.

Should a candidate that you think has talent still not be giving you what you are looking for, try to elicit her perceptions about the patient. Sometimes the reason an audition does not go well is because the candidate thinks you are looking for something other than what you really want. However, it might be that the candidate is volunteering a number of items on the checklist, and you want to call her attention to the importance of waiting for a specific question before giving checklist information. Or, it might simply be a matter of your needing to coach the candidate into expressing the patient's emotional tone in a different way.

Whatever the problem is with the portrayal, taking a few minutes to coach the candidate during the audition is invaluable. By doing so, you will get a more concrete sense of how it will be to work with the candidate during training. This is the kind of information that will make the final selection of your SPs a more informed process.
After coaching the candidate, do a short interview of the case again and see if the audition goes any better.

- *Have the candidate fill out the abridged checklist immediately after the audition interview.* Save all your conversation for after the SP has finished recording his responses on the checklist. (I suggest auditioning all cases with a checklist, even cases to be used in the teaching program. This gives you an idea of how good the candidate will be in carrying out the learning challenges built into the case. Thus, a specific audition can become a general audition for your needs in a future clinical skills examination.)

- *Audition candidates on complex physical simulations.* Generally speaking, if the simulation of the physical findings is simple—such as indicating that an area of the leg is mildly painful when touched—it is not necessary to take time for this during the audition. However, when cases call for more involved simulations, such as those requiring complicated neurological findings or the performance of a pneumothorax, auditioning the candidate's ability to perform these simulations is an essential part of the process.

Another reason to audition the candidate on the physical exam is if you are concerned about whether a given candidate might be troubled by being physically exposed or being in a patient gown during a clinical encounter. By having the SP go through this experience during the audition, both of you will get a better sense of whether the potential SP will be comfortable with this part of the encounter. It is often during the physical examination segment of the audition that certain necessities (that the candidate might not have heard in your verbal description) become clear, and issues arise, for example:

> One experienced SP, after going through the audition for an abdominal pain case that required the expression of intense pain throughout the encounter, decided the case was too stressful for him. Another patient discovered that she would have to remove her bra for a cardiac exam if the student asked her to.

Better to learn at this point in the recruitment process that a candidate is not comfortable with certain physical requirements than to find this out during training. Here is a rule of thumb: if there is any question about whether or not a candidate will be able to perform a particular simulation, audition it.

- *Compare the candidate's checklist with the one your assistant filled out during the audition.* The discussion you have with the candidate about missed items is as valuable as determining how accurate the candidate's responses are on the whole. Because the candidate will not have had the benefit of training to understand the specific meaning of each checklist item, it is important to let him explain how he understands an item that he missed—and why he did or did not give credit for that item. By working in this manner, you can learn how the candidates think, whether they interpret items with a broad understanding, or quite literally. It is also an opportunity to detect personality traits, such as whether the candidate is open to your suggestions, is defensive, or is insistent about his own interpretation.

- *If you still have mixed feelings about a candidate, talk with him before he leaves.* You can hold this conversation right after the audition in the same room. It can help you clarify in your own mind what your uneasiness is about the person, as the following example illustrates:

During one interview, a candidate's performance was so outstanding that I was sure he would be someone we would hire—until we went over his checklist. His recall was abysmal. He seemed to be an intelligent, thoughtful person, so I decided to talk with him about the surprising discrepancy in the two activities. In the brief discussion we had, he revealed that he had recently been under a lot of personal stress. This information and the general tone of our conversation made me feel it might be worth reauditioning him if the selection process warranted. Under other circumstances, we might have put his picture and resume in the casting file with a note to "hire only for teaching or demonstration work."

- *Thank the candidate for coming.* Always thank the candidates at the end of their audition and let them know when you anticipate getting back to them with the casting decisions. It shows your appreciation for the time they have spent trying out for you, and your respect for their natural concern over whether they will be chosen.

- *Debrief with your assistant about the candidates immediately after the audition.* Having a discussion on the merits of each prospective SP as soon as possible helps you crystallize details about the candidate's performance. You can do this after each candidate leaves, taking 5 minutes between auditions; or, if you wish to include the manager who has been observing the candidates in the waiting room, you can have a discussion about all the candidates at the end of the auditioning session.

- *Take performance notes.* In the comment section of each candidate's profile form, jot down the points about the person's audition that you want to remember. These immediate impressions are the essence of the process that is the audition. The elements of the audition about which to make notes have been discussed throughout this section, but to summarize, they might include observations about
  - the candidate's ability to take direction.
  - the realism of their performance.
  - why you would, or would not, like to work with this person.
  - the accuracy level of the checklist completed by the candidate.
  - which items were missed on the checklist (file the checklist with the candidate's Profile Form).
  - the thoughtfulness of the candidate's responses to any missed checklist items.

- *Start a "List of Top Candidates."* As soon as the first audition session is finished, begin keeping track of the candidates who have impressed you the most. You want to avoid having to review all the audition videos when it comes time to making your final choices. Make a list of the outstanding candidates, including brief notes on each person's notable qualities and start your photo mural. This should make your final selection process relatively effortless even if you have auditioned numerous candidates.

SELECTION

Even before selecting the best candidates for each of the cases, it is wise to establish a committee to help you make selection decisions along the way. Keep the selection committee small so that the decision making can take place in a timely fashion. The make-up of the committee can be as simple as the SP coach and an assistant who participated in the auditions, but it can also include consultants who can be called when questions arise. Remember that the committee does not always have to meet as a group. A call to a single consultant might be all that is needed in most circumstances, such as whether a potential SP who has a scar or a real medical condition will affect the challenge or standardization of the case. Members of the selection committee can also help arbitrate adjustments the SP coach might feel are necessary to make in the demographics of a case, such as using someone outside the specified age range, or substituting persons of a culture not defined in the case materials. These consultants can include individual members of the CPX advisory committee, other clinical faculty with a vested interest in the selection process, or the psychometrician responsible for the data analysis on the exam results.

A combination of calling on individual consultants, reviewing the audition videos, and brainstorming in committee can help you clarify virtually all issues that arise during selection. If, in addition, you have made a List of Top Candidates, the process should be a fairly smooth one.

Selection Principles

The following is a summary of the guidelines that will impact this final selection process.

- Hire candidates who best fit the demographics of the case.
- Try to select people with similar body types or physical appearance.
- Select as backup one candidate more than you will need.

- Hire persons who take direction well. Of course, consider high on the list those who performed the case believably without additional coaching, whose ability to simulate the physical findings was realistic, and who had a high level of accuracy in filling out the checklist. But should a given candidate fall short in these areas, the best criteria for success in training is the candidate's ability to hear what you suggest, and then adapt their performance to comply with what you want from the case.

- Hire people with whom you think you can get along. There is good reason to make this selection criterion as important as any of the others. You will be working intimately with each of the chosen candidates for an intense period of time—and they will be working in the same way with each other. This is why you want as harmonious and as flexible a group of SPs as you can find. Anyone, no matter how brilliant a performer, who insists on interjecting their interpretation of the case, or who simply talks too much, or in any way seems incompatible with your work style, is going to make training difficult for everyone.

- Try not to hire anyone out of desperation. Hiring someone you are ambivalent about is asking for problems. If you are unsure about a candidate, trust your uncertainty.

Strategy for Notifying the Candidates

It is my belief that everyone who has auditioned deserves a response. Even if your program is so large that it is impossible to call each person, I encourage sending a letter or, at least, an email officially letting each of the candidates know whether or not they have been selected. The key rationale for a personal response is respect for everyone who has shown an interest in your program and has participated in your recruitment process. This kind of thoughtfulness, along with honesty in letting the candidates know why they have not been chosen, goes a long way toward building the kind of relationships that will ensure satisfying collaborations and ultimately the success of your program. Once you have completed the selection process, here is a suggested strategy for contacting all the SPs who auditioned.

Procedure for Informing the Selected Candidates
- Call all the selected SPs first.
- Get verbal confirmation that each is still willing and available for training and performances. Do not assume that a candidate, who

was willing and able to participate in training and performances when he was at the audition, will necessarily be available by the time the selection process is complete.

- Find out each SP's availability during the week you want to schedule the first training sessions.

Procedure for Informing the Rejected Candidates

- Contact the SPs who have not been selected. Do this only *after* all the SPs who made the final cut have recommitted themselves to the project and to the first training session. It is better to wait before contacting those who were not your first choice; otherwise you might have to get in touch with one or another of them and rescind your original rejection because one of your primary choices was unable to accept your offer. As obvious as this seems, it is easy to make the mistake of sending final results to all the candidates in the excitement of at long last having cast a case.

What to Include in the Written Responses to all the Candidates

- *To the candidates whose performances and checklist accuracy were satisfactory.* This is the pool of candidates to whom you will turn should one of the selected SPs not work out. Therefore, the manner in which you let them know they have not been selected is very important. You want to be able to go back to these people and re-enlist them if necessary. Let them know that they were considered to be one of a handful of qualified candidates, but after the videos were reviewed, several others were chosen to perform the case for which they auditioned. Reassure them that their performance and checklist completion were satisfactory but that the final decisions were based on multiple factors. Let them know that other projects will be coming up throughout the year, that you have put their photograph and their SP Profile Form into your active file, and that you hope that you can work with them on another project in the future.

- *To the candidates whose performances were satisfactory, but whose checklist completion was marginal or unsatisfactory.* Let these candidates know that their performance was satisfactory but that there was concern about their ability to complete the checklists with a high enough level of accuracy. Tell them you are putting their photograph in the active file and that you hope they will be willing to work with you in the teaching program when an appropriate case comes up.

- *To the candidates whose performances and checklist accuracy were not satisfactory.* Thank the candidates for auditioning. Let them know that several other candidates were chosen to perform the case for which they auditioned. Thank them again for their time and interest in your program.

Postselection Procedures

All of the following should be done at least a week before the SPs' first training session:

- Select a date for the first training session that is compatible with the availability of all SPs performing the same case.
- Mail the following to the SPs so that they have these materials at least several days prior to your first meeting with them:
  - training materials, including the checklist and the guide to the checklist. (In the interest of exam security, do not send these materials electronically to the SPs.)
  - two copies of the Letter of Agreement.
  - a Recorded Image Consent-and-Release Form (see Appendix B3).

  Your cover letter accompanying these materials should let the standardized patients know that before the first training session you expect them
  - to be familiar with all the training materials.
  - to prepare a written list of their questions regarding the case.
  - to sign copies of the Letter of Agreement and Recorded Image Consent-and-Release Form.

Encourage the standardized patients to call you prior to the first training session if they have questions regarding the Letter of Agreement or the Consent-and-Release Form. You want to know about any non-training issues before you start working with the SPs. Although it does not happen often, occasionally an SP will get cold feet after seeing all the expectations clearly laid out in writing. If you become aware of this prior to the first training session, you will have an opportunity to dispel any doubts the SP may have, or if the SP decides not to participate, time to recruit another candidate from your selection list and still be on schedule with the training program.

The Letter of Agreement

This letter is not a legally binding document. It does, however, spell out in writing for the standardized patients what your expectations for them are

and what you and the SPs have agreed to verbally. The major components
of such a Letter of Agreement should include information on

- training:
  - number of training sessions.
  - general information on what will happen during each session.
  - total amount the SP will be paid for training.
- location for training, including parking arrangements.
- performances:
  - dates of the event for which the SP needs to be available.
  - the amount the SP is to be paid for training and for participation
    in each exam administration
- video recording of them during training sessions and review of
  their training performances by the CPX advisory committee. The
  SPs should be informed in writing that if their performances do
  not meet the standards of the advisory committee they may be
  terminated at any time during the process.
- ownership of patient cases (optional).
- statements requiring the SP's signature.
  - signed consent statement in which the SP agrees to all terms
    stated in the Letter of Agreement.
  - verification that the SP does not have contact with any of the
    examinees.

Recorded Image Consent-and-Release Form

Because video recording is an integral part of all training and performance
activities on any project having to do with clinical skills assessment, it is a
good idea to have the standardized patients sign a document that indicates
they have given their permission to be video recorded and that delineates
other purposes for which these recordings might be used.

When difficulties arise, they usually do so because the subjects were
not fully informed. Depending on your needs, it might be worthwhile
to create a consent-and-release form that is multipurpose (see sample in
Appendix B3). It is also important to inform the SPs that you will let them
know and get their approval first should anyone want to use the video
recordings for any purposes other than those stated in the document.

Last Details Before You Begin Training

Call all the SPs a day or two before the first training session to remind them
of the date and time you expect them. Remind them to bring their calendars to the first session in order to schedule the other training sessions.

Scheduling the training sessions when everyone is in the same room looking over their calendars together is much easier than trying to do this with each individual over the phone. In addition, your reminder phone call before the first training session is often a time when the SPs will share concerns with you. You can also remind them to review the documents you sent them earlier in preparation for the beginning of training.

CHAPTER SUMMARY

Because recruitment is of the utmost importance in the selection of SPs to portray the patient case, this chapter has provided extensive detail on

- recruitment principles, including kinds of persons to recruit to fit the patient case, backup policy, and candidates' desired qualities.
- recruitment resources, including outside agencies, recommendations from SPs, and publications.
- recruitment procedures, including when to start recruitment and the steps in the process of screening for potential candidates via telephone.
- auditioning principles and logistics, including when to initiate auditioning, optimum number of candidates to audition per session, requirements in personnel, hardware, and the physical layout of the environment.
- auditioning materials, including an SP profile form, casting aids, case summaries, and an abridged checklist.
- auditioning procedures for orientation and the audition itself.
- selection and notification of all of the candidates on their selection status.
- postselection activities, including mailing the selected SPs specific case documents to use in preparation for their first training session.

LOOKING AHEAD

All of the procedures for training the standardized patients are in the remaining chapters of Part Two. Chapter 6 introduces this part of the book with an overview of the training process. The following chapters are devoted to specific training protocols for each of the four training sessions and the Practice Exam. There is also a chapter on training options and variations.

Training the Standardized Patients: An Overview

In this part of the book you will find detailed procedures for training standardized patients to perform in any high-stakes clinical skills assessment. The preparation of standardized patients for such examinations requires the most rigorous form of performance training because these examinations have consequences that are decisive for the examinees: matriculating from second year to the intensive third year of clerkship training, graduating from medical school, or being granted a license to practice medicine. Our goal in preparing the SPs for performing in such clinical competency examinations is threefold: to ensure that all SPs

- arrive at seamless portrayals indistinguishable from actual clinical encounters with real patients. By the end of their training, the SPs should understand the patient so thoroughly that, no matter what comes up in the encounter, they can respond with the same internal consistency as the real patient might have done under the same circumstances.
- can provide the same challenge(s) for the medical student examinees.
- can demonstrate virtually flawless proficiency in delivering the facts and physical findings of the case, and on any post-performance tasks required of them, such as filling out checklists and giving effective feedback to the examinees.

GENERAL GUIDELINES FOR TRAINING

As you read through and use the procedures described in the next several chapters, remember that you can customize them for your particular needs

151

and for use in other circumstances (such as those found in chapter 11, Variations on the Training Sessions). Your decisions regarding the necessary amount and type of training depend on

- the situation (assessment versus teaching).
- the requirements of the SPs, that is, performance only; performance and verbal feedback; or performance, checklist, and written comments.
- the experience of the SPs.
- the abilities of the SPs.
- the number of SPs being trained.
- the difficulty of the patient case.
- the complication of the checklist or feedback protocols.

When deciding on how much or what kind of training the SPs need, a good rule of thumb to follow is *when in doubt, err on the side of more, rather than less, training.*

Training Principles

Having established these general guidelines, I offer the following principles for you to consider when training your SPs.

Keep in Mind the Distinct Set of Skills Required of Each SP

It is equally important for both the coach and the SPs to understand the six separate elements that go into making up a consummate standardized patient performance:

1. Realistic portrayal of the patient.
2. Appropriate and unerring responses to whatever the student says or does.
3. Accurate observation of the medical student's behavior.
4. Flawless recall of the student's behavior.
5. Accurate completion of the checklist.
6. Effective feedback to the student (written or verbal) on how the patient experienced the interaction with the student.

Make Sure That all of Your SPs Understand What Is Meant by Standardization

You may have decided to present the concept of standardization to the candidates initially during the auditioning process, but it is vital to have an in-depth conversation about what you mean by *standardized* patient with everyone who is embarking on training for the first time.

Standardization is often thought of in terms of *facts* and *behaviors*. But we know that standardization is more complex than this. Of course, the coach must ensure that there is (a) standardization of the facts—however, standardization in this area is not merely training an SP to accurately give the facts at the appropriate time in the encounter—though it is partly that and (b) standardization of behaviors. Because standardization does require training the SPs to perform specific behaviors when simulating *physical findings*, many believe it is also about prescribing *exact* behaviors that every SP must perform to express a given *emotion* or *psychological state*—which it is not. Not all behaviors in a patient portrayal need be exactly alike among the SPs. In fact, solidifying the behaviors, that is, requiring each person to perform exactly the same actions/reactions to express a given internal feeling state—for example, bouncing a leg or speaking fast without completing sentences at the opening of an encounter to show anxiety—often produces instead a performance that is read as phony (see p. 45: Blending Standardization With the Creative Process in chapter 3).

I suspect that some of the negative reactions that many in our field have about their experiences of working with actors are the result of (a) selecting the wrong person to portray the case, (b) failing to comprehend how actors perceive and approach their work, or (c) trying to standardize a case by requiring the SPs to incorporate the same pre-defined external behaviors into their emotional portrayals of the patient. What we are striving for in the standardization of an emotional or psychological condition is each SP's authentic portrayal of the patient's internal state so that anyone interacting with the SP will have the realistic cues needed to *perceive* the emotion as intended, despite the fact that each SP might behaviorally *express* the patient's emotion in various ways.

What this means is that we must work from the understanding that each human being is unique, that each SP has subtly distinct ways of expressing emotions that are naturally his own, and that these unique expressions of emotion, if realistically portrayed, will be perceived universally as what they are. This is how it is possible for each of us to read how someone else is feeling. Therefore, it is not necessary to force each SP into the same behaviors in order to ensure that the emotion of the patient he is portraying is universally understood. Knowing this, we can trust that if one SP more naturally portrays sadness, for example, by a flat affect and a slumping of the body, and another by lack of eye contact and heaviness of speech, both SPs will be perceived as portraying sadness so long as these manifestations are coming from an authentic place inside each of them.

Know What Standardization Means for SPs Who Have a Background in Acting

Trained actors are likely to consider standardizing a performance to be a negative concept. Skilled actors do not strive to interpret or perform a part the same way that anyone else does. In fact, when working on a part, they often avoid seeing other actors' performances, precisely in order not to be influenced by someone else's interpretation of the same character. Because actors do not usually work together as a team on a single role, as we do in our SP work, we must address this entirely different way of approaching the part of the patient or we might find ourselves dealing with resistance from the actors—and perhaps not know why.

The method of working toward standardization that I propose does not conflict with the actor's notion of discovering and embodying the characteristics of the patient through his own uniqueness of vision and talent. However, this is exactly what many actors anticipate when they hear the word *standardize*. This is why it is important for us to make sure our actor SPs understand the following:

- We want them to prepare and perform their cases in whatever way honors their skills in bringing the patient to life.
- What will be different about working on a standardized patient case is that all of us will be working collectively to come to a shared interpretation of the patient.
- That the intent of the case authors, coupled with the coach's insights into the case, are the necessary ingredients that must inform their process.

Once actors have worked together in a collaborative environment on an SP role, they generally grow to appreciate working in this mutually supportive way. In fact, they often get involved to the point that they begin to support one another with suggestions about each other's portrayals. This collective mission, guided by the coach's vision, is what we are striving for.

Train all the SPs Who Are Performing the Same Case Together, as a Group

Try to create among all the SPs a single-minded understanding of the patient: her affect, her needs, the facts of the case, and the interpretation of checklist items. Issues, concerns, and examples that come up in training are the very substance of this single-minded understanding of the case among all the SPs.

If we train the SPs separately, we not only create extra work for ourselves, but each SP also experiences growth in her understanding of the case in different ways, with different nuances. It is cumbersome, if not impossible, to remember all the insights that we and each SP discover during individual training, and then to share those insights with the other SPs every time we meet separately with them. Hence the need for training collectively.

Consider Carefully Whether You Want to Mix Actors With Non-Actors to Perform the Same Case

The training process can become needlessly difficult if we mix actors with non-actors on cases that have strong emotional elements—or other challenges requiring acting expertise—built into them. As we have seen, SPs of different skill levels require different methods of coaching. We dishonor the actors we have hired if we have to spend too much time during training working to bring a non-actor to their same level of performance. Unless the non-actor is a natural (that is, unselfconsciously able to tap into his own emotional resources), I suggest using non-actors primarily for cases that do not require manifestations of strong feelings. With such cases, the key requirement of the SP is the ability to be himself while delivering accurate information in a straightforward manner (see p. 9: Hiring Actors or Non-Actors as SPs, in chapter 1).

Hold to Your Vision of the Case While Allowing the SPs to Shape Their Portrayals Within Their Collective Understanding

It is the job of the coach to elicit a realistic portrayal from the SPs while allowing them to work in ways that are most natural for them. If we find that an SP's portrayal does not meet our criteria, then we need to share what we are experiencing and guide the SP into modifying her performances. In order to do this, we must have

- a clear understanding of who the patient is and how the patient should come across to the student.
- an ability to guide the SPs toward consensus in how everyone understands the patient.
- the capability of coaching each SP toward a portrayal that not only supports our vision but is integrated with the SPs' collective interpretation of the patient.

As their coach, our job is to create a safe environment that gives the SPs (actors and non-actors alike) space to shape their portrayals within that common vision. (For more details on coaching the SPs on performance, see chapter 3 on Acting and chapter 4 on Directing.)

Make Sure That a Clinician Who Is Unfamiliar With the Case Validates the Authenticity of the Trained SPs' Performances

Even if you as a coach have a background in clinical medicine, it is best to have a clinician who has not worked with the SPs on the case verify that they are performing it in an accurate and realistic manner. This authenticity check should take place at the stage in training when you feel confident that the SPs are prepared to perform the case. (In training for a CPX, this is usually the session just before the Practice Exam.) Any clinician who comes fresh to an encounter has the advantage of experiencing the patient for the first time, which allows inaccuracies and irregularities of performance to be more easily detected.

Schedule Refresher Training if an SP Has Not Performed the Case for 3 Weeks or Longer

Refresher training is a must under these circumstances because it is too easy to forget certain nuances—in performance, in the giving of feedback, and/or in checklist completion—when one has been away from the case for any length of time. Look at it this way: If an actor had rehearsed for a play, performed in it until the end of the run, then 3 weeks later performed in the play when it opened for another run—no producer or director would have taken a chance on letting the play go on without another rehearsal.

Limit Any Single Training Session to No More Than 3½ Hours

At times you may feel that your SPs need more practice than can be accomplished in a 3½-hour session. This is especially true if the case portrayal or the checklist is complicated. Resist the temptation, however, to extend a training session. The SPs' fatigue and their inability to concentrate will only bring diminishing returns. It is better to add an additional, perhaps shorter, session at another time.

Require the SPs to Use the Guide to the Checklist Every Time They Fill Out a Checklist After a Clinical Encounter

The guide to the checklist is a critical resource for improving and maintaining SP checklist accuracy. As you know, both during training and an actual exam, the SPs complete a checklist after every clinical encounter by recording what occurred during the interaction with the medical student. However, without the guide to the checklist, the SPs might be inclined (particularly when a question arises about a student's actions) to interpret the items on the checklist in their own way and by their own standards, which may not be what the case author or clinical faculty had in mind when they created the checklist. Therefore, in order to assure that the SPs understand the meaning of each item on the checklist in the same way, the guide must do the following:

- Make clear the *overall intent* of each checklist item. This is particularly important if the item itself has multiple facets or interpretations to it. In order to accurately determine when a student's behavior deserves credit, the SPs need a thorough understanding of what each item is designed to assess.
- Include *several examples* of the ways that examinees might fulfill the intent of the item.

Every student approaches the clinical encounter differently, whether it is the way she asks a question or makes a statement, or how she gives the patient information or performs the nuances of a physical examination maneuver. Sometimes the uniqueness of a medical student's style of eliciting information from a patient can confuse the SP when she is filling out the checklist after the encounter. If the guide contains examples of different approaches that students might take that warrant giving or not giving credit on a particular item, it helps the SPs grow in discrimination and accuracy when making their checklist decisions (see Appendix A5, Guide to the Checklist).

If the SPs become accustomed to using the guide during training, they are more likely during an actual exam to refer to it as a matter of course whenever they have a question about how to record what the medical student said or did.

One way to be sure that the SPs are using the guide to the checklist is to print it on colored paper so that it stands out from the checklist itself. This makes it easier for the SPs to find it and easier for you to be certain that they are using the guide when filling out the checklist. Even if your SPs are learning to use the checklist via computer and have an optional drop-down guide that explains each checklist item, it is still helpful to give the SPs a printed copy of the guide so that they can make notes, study these materials at home, and refer to their personalized copy when completing the checklist during CPX administrations.

Preview the Upcoming Training Session With the SPs

Make it a point at the end of each training session to preview the next session with the SPs. This gives them an idea of your expectations and guides them in their preparation.

Training Manuals

You will need a training manual for yourself and a training manual for each of your SPs. Three-ring binders work well for both because of the flexibility they provide for using the materials and for removing and adding various components during training.

The Coach's Training Manual

I recommend that the manual you use be divided into sections by the four training sessions and the Practice Exam. Each section should include the corresponding training session's Outline of the Training Procedures (OTP) and any other materials you have or will be handing out to the SPs, such as the Letter of Agreement, Recorded Image Consent-and-Release Form, the training materials, and any information you want the SPs to have regarding giving feedback. (See the box on the facing page for a sample of recommended contents for the coach's training manual.)

Outline of the Training Procedures to Include in Your Training Manual

On my Web site (www.coachingsps.com), you will find the Outline of the Training Procedures for the SP Coach's Training Manual. This detailed outline is intended for your use during the training sessions and should be part of your coach's manual. The remainder of the chapters in this section provide detailed, step-by-step training procedures that are outlined in the OTP, including the four training sessions and the Practice Exam. You can download the OTP from the Web site to put in your three-ring binder and use as a guide when you are working with your SPs during the training sessions. It can also serve as a summary of all the training procedures that are provided in this part of the book.

Layout of the Training Procedures

All of the materials in both the OTP for the coach's training manual and the information on each training session in the chapters that follow are organized by these categories:

1. *The Goal of the Training Session*—primary purpose of the session.
2. *Training Setting*—the physical environment for the training session.
3. *Summary of the Training Activities*—overview of each training session.

The Coach's Training Manual

Training Session One
- OTP for Training Session One
- Letter of Agreement
- Recorded Image Consent-and-Release Form
- Case Materials:
  - Presenting Situation and Instructions to the Student
  - Training Materials
  - Checklist (copy of electronic data collection software version)
  - Guide to the Checklist
  - Laboratory/diagnostic test/physical exam results (if needed)
  - Other information (including special equipment needed)

Training Session Two
- OTP for Training Session Two
- Checklist "keys" for each video recording to be shown

Training Session Three
- OTP for Training Session Three
- Cheat sheets for practice interviews (if needed)
- General information and principles on giving feedback
- Guidelines for giving written feedback
- List of feedback descriptors

Training Session Four
- OTP for Training Session Four
- Guidelines for the SPs on the Practice Exam

The Practice Exam
- OTP for the Practice Exam
- Guidelines for the SPs on the CPX

In addition, the coach should have enough blank checklists available for everyone's use throughout training, from Session Two through the Practice Exam.

---

4. *Reminders*—reminders of the coach's tasks (such as handing out new materials, going over administrative details with the SPs, etc.) and reminders for the SPs.
5. *Session Training Activities*—a detailed explanation of the training activities.

6. *Preparation of the SPs for the Next Session*—preview of the up-coming session.
7. *The Coach's Preparation for the Next Session(s)*—what the coach needs to do between sessions.

The SPs' Training Manual

The SPs' manual (see the following box) should include everything you have in your coach's manual except the Outline of the Training Procedures and a few coaching aids. If there is enough time between the final selection of the SPs and the first training session, it is beneficial to send the training materials portion of their manual to the SPs before they meet with you, along with the Recorded Image Consent-and-Release Form and the Letter of Agreement. SPs appreciate being able to take a preliminary look at the patient case they will be portraying. To help them prepare for the start of training, you can request that they write down any questions that arise while they are studying the materials and bring them to the first training session.

The SPs' Training Manual

Letter of Agreement (two copies)
Recorded Image Consent-and-Release Form

Case Materials:
    Presenting Situation and Instructions to the Student
    Training Materials
    Checklist (copy of electronic data collection software version)
    Guide to the Checklist
    Laboratory/diagnostic test/physical exam results (if needed)
    Other information (including special equipment needed)

General information and principles on giving feedback
Guidelines for giving written feedback
List of feedback descriptors

Guidelines for the SPs on the Practice Exam

Guidelines for the SPs on the CPX

CHAPTER SUMMARY

This chapter has provided an overview of the training of the standardized patients who have been selected to perform the CPX cases including

- general guidelines for determining the amount of training necessary.
- training principles for working with the SPs.
- recommended contents for the coach's and the SPs' training manuals and an introduction to the Outline of the Training Procedures (OTP) which can be downloaded for inclusion in the SP Coach's Manual. The OTP can be found at www.coachingsps.com

LOOKING AHEAD

Table 6.1 on the next page gives an overview of the four training sessions and the Practice Exam, which are conducted with the SPs in preparation for performing as standardized patients in the CPX. With this overview, the OTP, and your training manual in hand, you will be ready to start working with your SPs in earnest.

Note: The OTP on www.coachingsps.com provides a more detailed outline of the training sessions and the Practice Exam than this brief overview in Table 6.1.

Table 6.1 Overview of the SP Training Sessions Leading to the CPX

Training Session	Purpose	Estimated Time
Session One: Familiarization With the Case (Chapter 7)	-Coach introduces the checklist and the guide to the checklist and gives overview of case materials. -SPs read through training materials together. -View video of student/SP encounter (if *new* SPs are being trained). -Do progressive interview with the SPs with coach in role of medical student.	3 hours
Session Two: Learning to Use the Checklist (Chapter 8)	-Do brief progressive interview with coach in role of the medical student. -Practice using the checklist and the guide to the checklist.	3 hours
Session Three: Putting It All Together (Performance, Checklist, Feedback) (Chapter 9)	-Introduce SPs to exam room etiquette. -Do two practice encounters with each SP stressing 1. authenticity and standardization of performance. 2. accuracy of performance and checklist use. 3. writing effective feedback.	3.5 hours
Session Four: The First Dress Rehearsal Clinician Verification of SPs' Authenticity (Chapter 10)	-First dress rehearsal and final training session. -Uninitiated clinician verifies SPs' performance authenticity by engaging in practice encounters in role of student. -Coach and nonperforming SPs observe performances from the monitoring room.	3 hours
Training Options: Variations on the Training Sessions (Chapter 11)	-The coach can vary the training sessions according to the case complexity, SPs' needs/experience. -Sessions can be added, combined, or reduced in number.	Varies by purpose of the training session
Practice Exam: The Final Dress Rehearsal (Chapter 12)	-"Mock exam" with participation of all SPs and all administrative support staff. -Residents serve as examinees to pilot the exam logistics; gives SPs a sense of how the CPX will run and coaches a chance to give SPs final feedback.	Varies by number of cases
The CPX: (The Actual Exam)	-Medical students meet and interview individual SPs in examining rooms during an actual exam while rotating through patient cases. -Coaches/faculty observe clinical encounters from monitoring room. -SPs fill out checklists, write feedback then following the exam debrief with coach and/or faculty.	Varies by number of cases

CHAPTER SEVEN

Training Session One: Familiarization With the Case

During Training Session One, you and the standardized patients will begin to get to know one another and the patient case that all of you will be working on together for the next month or so. The SPs will have an opportunity to read through the training materials as a group and start their own individual process of coming to know the patient they will be portraying, as well as some of the other performance requirements that will be expected of them.

The Goal of Training Session One

The purpose of Training Session One is to familiarize the SPs with all of the training materials and to give them an initial experience of performing the patient case during a progressive interview, as well as a chance to practice simulating the physical findings under your guidance.

The Training Setting

This session should take place in two areas—a small conference room for the read-through of the training materials and the progressive interview as well as an examination room where you and the SPs can participate in the demonstration/practice of the physical findings.

Summary of the Training Activities

You will be supervising the SPs' review of the training materials, introducing them to the checklist and the guide to the checklist, and—if any

SPs are new to this work—showing them a medical student/SP encounter on video. All of the SPs will participate in a progressive interview of the entire case with you (the coach) assuming the role of the medical student interviewer. You will also introduce the SPs to all of the physical findings, demonstrate those that they will need to simulate, and give them a chance to practice producing those simulated findings.

Reminders

Collect the Signed Recorded Image Consent-and-Release Form and a Copy of the Letter of Agreement

Before training starts, collect from the SPs these two documents that were included with the training materials you sent them prior to this first training session. Encourage them to keep their copy of the Letter of Agreement with their training manual as a reference to use throughout the training. This letter is not a legally binding document, but having your expectations in writing, signed by the participants, makes clear the duties and responsibilities everyone has agreed on.

Discuss Parking Arrangements for Training Sessions and Exam Performances

Parking can be one of the most frustrating logistical matters. If your SPs are tense or late to training sessions or performances, the quality of their participation is affected.

Go Over Performance Dates, Backup Policy, and "On Call" Requests

One last time, go over the inclusive dates of all performances, including the Practice Exam. Make sure that everyone understands that the program they are about to embark on must become a priority, especially now that they are about to start training.

Go over the backup policy and on call requests (see chapter 5 for details). Remember, you are going to train everyone as regularly performing SPs. No one is an understudy. If you use this method, all of the SPs will have the same level of training and performance experiences so that they are ready to cover for each other in an emergency.

Review Calendars and Schedule the Rest of the Training Sessions

Now that you have all the SPs who are performing the same case in a room together, go over your calendars and schedule the remaining training sessions. Try to schedule each session about 1 week apart to give the SPs time to process the work of the previous session and to prepare for the activities of the next. Only under extreme circumstances should you schedule two sessions any closer than 24 hours apart. Each training session is designed to build toward integration of the whole, so if you combine two sessions of the same case in a single day, it short circuits the personal integration each SP needs before taking on new material or moving on to the next level of mastery.

I discourage scheduling training for one SP on separate occasions from the others. There might not be a way around this for a single session if there is a scheduling problem. However, if it looks as if you will need to do separate training for more than one session, consider letting the person with the scheduling problem go, and recruit the next person on your List of Top Candidates. (This does not apply to working separately—beyond the required collective training—with individual SPs who need extra coaching to improve their performances.)

Inform the SPs That all Performances During Training Will Be Video Recorded for Review by the CPX Advisory Committee

Even though the SPs will already have signed a consent-and-release form agreeing to be recorded, it is wise to let them know verbally that every performance they do will be video recorded, from the first progressive interview in Training Session One to their final performance in the actual exam, the CPX. This is a good time to remind the SPs about the CPX advisory committee whose job it is to maintain the high standards that help to make the clinical assessment a reliable measure of the examinee's clinical competence. (The CPX committee only needs to review the training videos if you are concerned about a particular SP's performance.)

Remind the SPs of the Protocol Regarding Dismissal

Let the SPs know that anyone may be let go at any time during training or during the actual exam, if their performances and checklists are not up to CPX committee standards. This is a necessary discussion to have *before* the start of training. At some point in your career as an SP coach, you will be faced with the difficult task of removing someone from your roster of performers. Hopefully, it will be clear early on in the training that a particular person is not performing up to standard, but you might need to remove someone as late as during the CPX itself.

When you remind the SPs about this protocol, do it in a matter of fact, straightforward manner. Let them know that you are not telling them this to intimidate them and that, in fact, based on their auditions, you expect everyone to be able to perform up to standard.

Distribute the Training Manuals and Give the SPs an Overview of the Contents

If you expect your SPs to practice between training sessions (and you should), for exam security purposes I suggest not giving them electronic copies of the training materials. Using three-ring binders works well for the training manuals because you can add and remove items as needed during training. If the guide to the checklist is on colored paper, the SPs can find this document more easily when they want to make personal notations on it throughout the training. Let the SPs know that they are expected to bring their personal copy of the guide to the checklist with them to use at every exam administration, even if there is a guide already built into the electronic checklists that the SPs will be filling out. Give an overview of what is included in their training manuals so that they have an idea of what will be happening over the course of training.

Address the Confidential Nature of the Materials in the Training Manual

Several years ago, an incident occurred that illustrates how important it is to impress on the SPs the sensitive nature of the materials in their possession. Late one afternoon, a cashier called the standardized patient office asking if one of us had left a notebook in the medical school cafeteria. That "notebook" turned out to be a training manual that one of the SPs had inadvertently left behind after getting coffee following a training session!

Sometimes SPs, especially if they are new to your program, have not thought about the fact that all of the materials they are working with are secure examination materials and that if any of the medical students were to get their hands on them, the data from the case, and potentially the exam itself, would be compromised.

Session One Training Activities (Estimated Time: 3 hours)

Because most of this session is devoted to familiarization with the training materials and other documents in the training manuals, the best location to do this work is in a small conference room with a table around which you and the SPs can sit facing one another with enough room to comfortably lay out the training manuals. The progressive interview, which you will do later in this session, can also be done in the conference room.

However, your demonstration of the physical examination and the simulated physical findings will need to be done in one of your larger clinic rooms.

Review the Training Materials With the SPs

Have the SPs Remove the Checklist from the Three-Ring Binder

If the SPs have the checklist next to the training materials so that they can easily refer to it while they are reading through the materials, you can call their attention to each checklist item as it relates to the section of the training materials you are working on. It also helps the SPs to see what the relationship is between the facts of the case, what they are allowed to volunteer, and what they must hold back in order to maintain the integrity of the checklist.

Have the SPs Read Through the Training Materials Together Out Loud

Even though the SPs might have received the training materials prior to this session, it is still essential to have them read through them again together. If you simply ask the SPs if they have any questions, you may not get to all of the issues they might have, even if they followed your directive to write down questions while studying the materials ahead of time.

By going through the materials out loud together—sharing the reading equally among the SPs—everyone is thinking about the details of the case together in the moment. As each person reads, listens, shares his thoughts, and asks questions, insight about the patient grows in an atmosphere of mutual discovery. It is a much more thorough way to make sure that everyone understands the materials in the same way.

Once you have finished reading through the case together, ask the SPs one by one to tell you in their own words one of the following:

- What they understand about the patient.
- What the circumstances of the clinical encounter are and what the patient's attitude is toward the visit.
- What the patient wants or needs from the doctor during the encounter.
- What one mental image, feeling, or attitude has occurred to the SP about the patient.
- What the mood of the clinical encounter is (relaxed, tense, confrontational, etc.).

After you have heard the SPs' responses to these items, refer them to the case summary under the section "From the Patient's Perspective" at the end of the checklist (see Appendix A4, Checklist). This is the place where the SPs will write feedback about the interaction they had with the medical student. (For details on giving feedback, see Training Session Three in chapter 9.) If such a summary presenting the patient's point of view does not already exist in your checklist, you can create one, or you and your SPs can create one together while you are analyzing the training materials with them during this first session. If you already have such a summary, you can use it to engage the SPs in a discussion of their interpretation of the patient, get feedback from them on what they think might need adjusting in the summary, or ask them what else they think should be included. The summary can then be modified and used as a touchstone throughout the training to focus the SPs on a uniform interpretation of the case—which they participated in creating.

Here is an example of how relevant material (which came out of one such set of SP discussions) can be produced for writing the from-the-patient's-perspective summary. The patient case in this example is a 17-year-old named Brittany Eisler. One of the key issues the medical students need to address with her is the fact that, although Brittany is using birth control pills, she is otherwise having unprotected sex. The following are several concerns the young women performing this case felt were important from the point of view of Brittany:

- She would be open to suggestions like teen counseling, but only if the medical student helped her find a counselor without her parents knowing.
- She is already worried about the potential for getting HIV and other sexually transmitted diseases so she does not need a lecture from the student telling her what she already knows and is concerned about.
- She needs help in how to raise the subject of condom use with her boyfriend. One of the young female SPs portraying Brittany phrased it this way: "I love Sean. I'm not going to stop having sex with him no matter how much the student doctor tells me not to. What I need is help in how to bring the subject of condoms up with him."

The written training materials are a detailed blueprint, a framework of the patient case within which the SPs will improvise during each encounter. But it is the coach's verbal elaboration and the discussion among the SPs that will help them gain insight into the patient case in the way that each new set of SPs needs to do when beginning the process of training. It is this expansion of understanding who-the-patient-is that makes training interesting and keeps the process fresh.

The coach must be ready to discuss his perception of the patient, but he must also be ready to incorporate any ideas from the SPs that build on the essence of the case. This is how to keep the case alive. Each time you train someone to do the same case, it will be slightly different, but the case will remain standardized because you will be protecting the core interpretation. It is your thorough understanding of the patient case and the purpose for which it is being used, as well as the particular challenges to the medical student that are built into the case, that will allow you the freedom to work with the SPs in the manner that I am suggesting.

Document any Inconsistencies or Problems With the Training Materials

While reading the training materials, note any changes or additions that would make the materials clearer or more complete. Incorporate these changes into the original as soon as possible so that you can give the SPs updated pages at the next session. Do not let the SPs work solely from their own notes because each may have interpreted the discussion differently. The point is to develop consensus on their understanding of the patient so that they come across in the same realistic way and present the same challenge to each of the students, no matter which of them is playing the case.

Introduce the SPs to the Guide to the Checklist

A general introduction to the guide to the checklist is enough for this session. Emphasize the guide's importance in assisting them to interpret each of the checklist items in the same way. In preparation for the next session, ask the SPs to carefully study the guide and make notes next to any item that is unclear to them.

View a Medical Student/SP Encounter on Video (if You Have Any Trainees New to Standardized Patient Work)

Make sure the SPs understand why you are showing them the video. Viewing an encounter on video is an excellent means of orienting *new* SPs to what they can expect during training and the CPX. SPs who have not done this kind of work before usually have questions about the environment in which they will be working, how the medical students will act, and what will happen during a clinical encounter. Watching one portrayal of their case on video usually answers these questions and dispels some of the anxiety they may have. However, I have concern about the value of this kind of video use for any other purpose. It is my belief that model videos are not the best means of standardization because these recordings can foster rote, lifeless performances, particularly if the purpose is for the SPs to mimic what they see in the model. If this is what standardization means, then there is no room for each SP to discover what he or she can bring to the requirements of the case. Indeed, training to a recorded performance can force the process into a rigidity that is not necessary for standardization. In short, I believe that the best training experience is a more fluid, interactive process than what is dictated by using a video recording as the means of standardization. (See p. 45: Blending Standardization With the Creative Process in chapter 3 for more on this subject.)

If you are showing a video for the benefit of the SPs who are new to this work, the SP's performance on the video recording must be impeccable. If there are any errors in the standardized patient's recorded performance, it can be harmful to the SPs watching the video, especially at this early stage of training. Even though you are not using this as a standardization tool, you do not want new trainees to learn bad habits from flawed performances on video; otherwise, you will have to spend valuable time trying to repair the SPs' impressions of the performance (and the specific errors) that the SPs absorbed while watching the video.

Do a Progressive Interview With all the SPs, Having Them Portray the Patient in Tandem

The progressive interview is a training technique that will help you and your SPs discover how close (or how remote) each person's interpretation of the patient is to that of the other SPs—and to your own expectations. (The progressive interview is the only activity that needs to be video recorded during this session.) By the time you get to this point in the training session, considerable discussion of the case has taken place and everyone usually feels that they understand the case and the patient. The next step is to give the SPs an opportunity to "try on" the patient, to see what he or she feels like *in performance.*

Before doing the progressive interview, describe the process to the SPs and remind them that the purpose of this exercise is to help them work as a team toward the goal of standardization—performing the case as if they were of one mind. Be sure that the SPs understand that, until the first dress rehearsal, you do *not* expect a finished performance every time they portray the case. Rather this is a time of exploration.

The physical set up for the progressive interview is important. The SPs should be sitting next to one another in a semicircle away from the conference table so that they have enough room to move and the freedom to express any body language that arises during this exercise. As the coach, you should face all the SPs directly so that a mere look from you is the cue that the SP is "on." Encourage the SPs to either look at you or look slightly downward so that they can maintain a connection with both you and their own internal process. If they look directly at the SP engaged in the interview with you (which is what they will be inclined to do), they will be drawn out of their own process into observing someone else's.

The progressive interview is just what the name implies. The coach, playing the part of the medical student, interviews each SP, one after the other, as the clinical encounter progresses from beginning to end. With this method, none of the SPs does a complete encounter. Instead, the coach engages one SP who continues the encounter where the previous one left off—as if she were the same person (patient). While one SP is being interviewed directly by the coach, the other SPs are actively, but silently, experiencing whatever is going on with the patient being interviewed. Their silent, active engagement should be so focused that when the coach looks to someone else to continue the interview, the next SP can pick up the responses, the affect, the feeling tone wherever the previous SP left off—as if she were the same person who had just been engaged in dialogue with the coach.

Let me give an example of what I mean by *silent, active engagement*. Suppose, at a given point in the encounter, the SP being directly interviewed by the coach starts to cry (as indicated in the training materials). So close to that feeling should the other SPs be, that were the coach to call on another SP, that SP would be able to continue the interview without a break in mood or emotion, perhaps even to the point of being on the edge of tears herself.

The progressive interview reveals the similarities and differences in interpretation of the case among the SPs. You can now begin to coach the SPs into the kind of performances you are looking for. The SPs will leave the session having discovered more accurately what it is that you want from each of them in performing the case and will therefore know specifically what each needs to work on in the interim before the next session. One of the most common discoveries that SPs make is how easy it is to volunteer information that is on the checklist, particularly when asked an open-ended question during the interview. An actor, who was amazed at her own performance during a progressive interview, said, "I've been doing improvisations all my life, but I've never had to remember what *not* to say." The progressive interview is always full of beneficial surprises.

At this point you might be asking some of the following questions about the progressive interview:

- *How long should each portion of the progressive interview last?* Do enough of the encounter to get a feel for how each SP is interpreting the patient. There are natural breaks in every encounter. As you work with this technique, you will instinctively sense when there is a logical place in the interview to move on to the next SP.

- *Should I interview the SPs in any particular order?*
  Do not go in the order in which the SPs are sitting. Mix it up. This keeps them more engaged because they do not know which SP you will call on to continue the interview.

- *What if there is a particularly difficult section of the interview? How will I know if all of the SPs can perform it acceptably well and in the same way?*
  There is no reason why a portion of the progressive interview cannot be repeated and thus replayed by each of the SPs. This is particularly important for the difficult emotional sections of an encounter. I encourage you to have each SP repeat one by one any section requiring an emotional response.

- *What if an SP interprets a segment of the encounter differently than I intend?*
  If the SP's interpretation is not what you are looking for, coach the person into the performance you envision. You may take a time out and stop the progressive interview at any point. One of the best reasons to take a time out is to coach the SPs into more of the kind of patient portrayal you want from them. One of the worst reasons to call a time out is to do more intellectualizing about the patient case. Now is the time for talk to be put into the service of action.

Another way to deal with an unacceptable performance—especially if you cannot articulate exactly what is not working—is to repeat that section of the progressive interview and have someone else play the patient to see if another SP's interpretation is closer to what you want. This process will often trigger an idea about why the previous portrayal was off. Then you can go back and work on it with the other SP.

Review the Simulated Physical Exam Findings Required by the Patient Case

During the first training session, the SPs need to be thoroughly oriented to all of the maneuvers on the checklist that are related to the physical examination (PE), *especially* those that require the patient to simulate a physical finding. Included in the physical examination section of the training materials should be a detailed, written description of all the physical exam maneuvers found in the checklist and how to simulate the physical findings, as well as any other commonly anticipated maneuvers the students might perform that are not on the checklist. If assessment of the student's performance on a given physical exam maneuver includes specific locations on the anatomy (such as where the medical student should place the stethoscope, or where the patient is experiencing certain neurological deficits), then diagrams of the patient's anatomy should also be included.

If you are just starting out as a coach and do not have a background in clinical medicine, when you are faced with coaching a new patient case that requires a physical examination or is based on a medical problem you have not worked with before, always try to get a clinician to go through the case with you before you start training. (See chapter 2, Clinical Skills: Acquiring the Basic Doctoring Skills, for suggestions on how to prepare yourself to train the physical examination.)

Prepare the SPs for the Physical Findings' Demonstration and Practice

Following the progressive interview, ask everyone to reconvene in an examination room for a demonstration of the physical findings. Make sure that the SPs understand the purpose of this physical exam session. Describe to the SPs the demonstration-and-practice session you have planned, in which you assume the role of the medical student examining the patient:

- Demonstrate on one of the gowned SPs all parts of the PE that are on the checklist.
- Encourage all the other SPs to gather around the examination table so that they can clearly see what you are doing. Urge them to ask questions about anything they do not understand.
- Verbally describe in detail each of the maneuvers, such as listening with a stethoscope and percussing the patient's lungs, as you are performing them.
- Have all the SPs locate the item on the checklist that corresponds to the maneuver you are demonstrating so that they begin to visualize where the items are located on the checklist.
- Demonstrate the *simulated* physical findings on the gowned volunteer; then have this SP practice them with you, in front of the others, until he can perform them correctly.
- Have each of the SPs, in turn, go through all of the simulatedfindings with you, especially those that are the more difficult to perform. (Thedifficult-to-simulate findings are the ones on which you auditioned the candidates.Therefore, you should feel confident that the SPs can perform these simulations. Going overthem with each of the SPs at this point in the training reinforces how to accuratelyportray the simulations so that they can practice them properly between sessions until theybecome second nature to them.)

If there is time, demonstrate the other physical exam maneuvers that the medical students might do that are *not* on the checklist so that the SPs feel prepared to deal with the unexpected.

In summary, regarding the physical exam findings, you should feel confident by the end of this session that your SPs know the following:

- What to expect in a physical exam.
- How to convincingly simulate the required physical findings.
- How to relate the PE maneuvers to the appropriate checklist item.
- What constitutes the proper performance of the maneuver.

Preparation of the SPs for Training Session Two

The SPs will need to practice their portrayals between this session and the next. Although there will be a short progressive interview at the beginning of the next training session in order for you to touch base with how the SPs are doing on their performances, most of Session Two is devoted to training the SPs in how to use the checklists that they fill out after each clinical encounter. The focus will be on checklist accuracy. Here are some suggestions to help the SPs prepare for the next training session.

Ask the SPs to Do a Number of Interviews With a Partner Between Sessions

Ideally, their partners would be one of the other SPs performing the case, but it can be anyone who is willing to help. Encourage the SPs to contact each other to practice before the next session. If the SP's partner is someone who is not familiar with the process, suggest that the SP create a list of questions from the training materials that his partner can ask him.

Help the SPs Prepare for the Work They Will Be Doing on the Checklists

Once the SPs feel reasonably familiar with the case portrayals, they should focus on reviewing the checklist and the guide to the checklist, making notes on anything they do not understand.

Let the SPs know that in the next session they will watch video recordings of real clinical exam performances of their case with several different students. They will be filling out checklists and going over them together. The focus of these viewings will be for the SPs to have a chance to observe real medical students in action, giving them an opportunity to make checklist decisions based on what they have perceived in the student's actual performances. Showing these videos is not meant as a device to demonstrate specifics of how you want the SPs to perform the case. In fact, selection of the videos for checklist training should not only consist of a variety of student styles and levels of expertise, but also ought to demonstrate how a variety of SPs' performances can be different and still produce accurate, realistic, standardized portrayals.

The Coach's Preparation for Training Sessions Two and Four and the Practice Exam

In addition to preparing for Session Two, at this time you will also need to plan ahead for Session Four and the Practice Exam.

Make Checklist "Keys" for the Videos You Will Use in Session Two

You need to have some standard to determine which answer is correct on every item of the checklist for each video-recorded student/SP encounter you show the SPs during the next practice session. The best way to handle this is to create a key ahead of time by filling out a checklist for each encounter while watching the video performances—rewinding whenever necessary to be sure that your answers are correct.

It is also a good idea to *make notes on your checklist key*, indicating what the student interviewer said or did that caused you to mark each item the way you did. You can then use these notes to respond to the SPs whenever there is a discrepancy in their checklist answers.

Start Recruiting Clinicians for Training Session Four

Now is a good time to start thinking about enlisting clinicians who are unfamiliar with the cases and who can verify that each SP is performing in a realistic manner during the first dress rehearsal, which takes place in Training Session Four. It is often challenging to find clinicians who are available for this activity at the time that is convenient for all of the SPs. The closer it gets to the final training session, the more difficult it becomes to find a clinician. So begin recruiting clinicians no later than at the end of this session or as soon as you have scheduled Training Session Four.

Here are some considerations for recruiting clinicians:

- *The kind of clinician to recruit.* The clinician you recruit to assist you in the final training session will depend on the type of case and the purpose of your clinical exam. Because the CPX is a clinical examination designed to assess medical students' abilities with general, commonly seen patient problems, a primary care physician (family physician, gynecologist, internist, or pediatrician) would be a good choice.

Be careful about asking specialists to participate in the final training session on a primary care examination. Specialists' expectations are different from those of primary care physicians. However, when preparing to give a specialty exam involving SPs, it is wise to have ongoing consultations with an appropriate specialist throughout case development and training—for example, to have an experienced geriatrician as a consultant on an exam designed to assess the clinical skills of geriatric residents.

- *The protocol for recruiting clinicians.* When recruiting the clinicians for Session Four, you can share the type of case and the presenting symptoms of the patient, but no other information about the case. Let her know that her participation will be focused on verifying that each SP who will be performing the case is portraying the patient in a realistic manner. Let her know that what you need from her, as an experienced clinician, is an assessment of whether the SPs come across as real as the patients she sees in her own practice. Make sure she knows that it is not *her* performance that is being assessed, and that if she wishes, she can even work with the SPs as if she were a medical student or resident. (For more details on what the clinician will be doing with the SPs, see Training Session Four in chapter 10.)

Start Recruiting Residents for the Practice Exam

As with the early recruitment of clinicians for Training Session Four, it is wise at this time to also begin recruitment of residents to participate in the Practice Exam as the examinees (taking the place of the medical students who will be the examinees in the actual CPX) during this final dress rehearsal, which is given just prior to the CPX itself. In essence, the Practice Exam is an opportunity for everyone on the CPX administrative team to rehearse the exam logistics, and for the SPs to experience more closely what the CPX will be like in terms of bringing the full force of their concentration to bear on performing their case multiple times, one after another with different examinees.[1]

---

[1] Note: The Practice Exam (which is a mock-up of the CPX) and all the administrations of the CPX should already have been scheduled before recruitment was started. There should be at least two days between the Practice Exam and the first administration of the actual CPX. This allows enough lead time to refine administrative procedures, work with SPs or staff who might be having difficulties with their assignments, and make other staffing decisions based on what has been observed.

NOTES TO THE SP COACH ABOUT
TRAINING SESSION ONE

During the first training session you will get your first impressions of how well your SPs are interacting with each other (that is, becoming members of a team), how responsive each is to your suggestions and analysis of the training materials, how well they are able to adapt their notions about the patient to the team's consensus, how well they are able to put those collective interpretations into play in their performances in the progressive interview, and, finally, how capable they are of taking direction from you on their portrayals and in producing the simulated physical examination findings. If you should find problems in any of these areas with any of your SPs, now—not later—is the time to deal with them. To that end, you might find the following suggestions helpful.

Ways to Deal With Behavioral or Performance Problems

If you have carefully auditioned your candidates, there should be no surprises in the performance capabilities of your SPs, but despite our best efforts, sometimes there are. Where you will first get a sense of this is from the progressive interview.

However, sometimes there are surprises in areas for which the audition was not meant to be used as a screening tool. The most frequent discovery usually has to do with the way the SP interacts with you or with the other trainees. Perhaps an SP challenges or resists your interpretation of the patient case, or is argumentative with the other SPs.

Recognize Any Tendency You Have to Avoid
Problematic Situations

When facing a potentially difficult situation with an SP, the most common instinct most of us have for dealing with it is avoidance. Avoidance can be present in any of the following guises:

- Wanting to ignore the situation (a common favorite).
- Talking ourselves into believing that our own perceptions are wrong (a close second).
- Hoping the SP will somehow magically be better the next time he comes.
- Feeling trapped because we have made a bad decision and do not have any backups who can take his place for the case.

Recognizing that we are avoiding an SP's behavioral or performance problem is the first step toward resolving it. As with so many other situations, the longer we wait the worse it gets, so it is best to deal with your concerns as soon as you become aware of them.

After the session, when all the other SPs have gone, spend a few minutes talking in private with the SP in question. If the issue is his behavior, try to find out whether or not he is aware of how he is coming across. If your concern is with his performance, ask him how he feels the progressive interview went for him.

Below are a few suggestions on how to approach working with such an SP. In Training Session Three (chapter 9), there is a section devoted to feedback that you might want to look at because the same principles of giving good feedback apply here, just as they do when the SPs or the faculty are sharing their observations on a medical student's behavior or performance with them. In coaching the SPs, we should be modeling the behavior we expect them to embody once they have been trained to give feedback to the students.

- Elicit the SP's perspective.
- Share what you have observed.
- Let the SP know what your expectations are.
- Together discuss ways the SP might improve the situation.

If the problem is behavioral, encourage the SP to reflect on the issues you *both* have identified and negotiate with him specific ways to modify the behaviors. If the SP has been challenging you on the interpretation of the case, and he does not improve his behavior substantially by the next session, consider letting him go. SP behavioral problems can occupy much of your energy and destroy the camaraderie among the SP team, which in turn can affect the whole training process.

Determine the Nature of the Performance Problem

If the problem is a performance issue, find out if the SP has any ideas about how she might work on the areas that are giving her difficulty. If she does not, offer some suggestions that she can try before the next session. If the performance problem is the SP's inability to realistically express the affect of the patient, the method for helping her will depend on the specific problem she is having. (See chapter 3 on Acting and chapter 4 on Directing to address performance issues.)

On the one hand, one reason that an actor's emotional portrayal might not be what you had in mind could stem from her needing more time to work through the material, more time to process the information from the training session before her performance reflects what you are looking for.

On the other hand, if a *non*-actor's performance is not what you anticipated, it might mean that you will need to get more involved with her early on. The non-actor's range of performance skills is limited compared to that of a competent trained-actor. The non-actor will potentially need more time, support, and coaching from you, with clear feedback about her performance, each step of the way.

If any performance issues uncovered in the progressive interview are of enough concern, you may want to have an additional training session with the SP. Let her know what you are thinking about before she leaves this training session. Schedule a time before the next session to do a practice interview with her, separate from the group. This might mean an extra $1/2$ hour to 1 hour of your time, but it will provide the reassurance you need to decide whether to keep the SP or to let her go.

Techniques for Assisting the SPs in Improving Their Performances

These methods can be helpful for all the SPs, not just for those having problems.

A Suggestion for Amplifying the SPs' Understanding of the Patient

Encourage the SPs to *live as the patient*. If the SP is not an actor, or has never prepared for a role, living as the patient can be one of the most effective tools for deepening his understanding of the patient. Encourage the SP to incorporate the patient's life into his own whenever he thinks of it before the next training session.

Based on details from the case, suggest that the SP imagine himself as the patient and do some of the things the patient does in his daily life. For example, the SP could ask himself: What does the patient do on waking? What is his morning routine? What does he have for breakfast? Does he go to work? If so, while driving to work, what is the patient thinking about—what is he concerned about? When he gets out of work, where does he go, what does he do? Encourage the SP to literally do the things he thinks the patient does, such as go to a gym, take a walk, or meet friends for a drink—and urge him to try to interact with the people he meets along the way *as if he were the patient!* And what about when he comes home? What is his home life like? What does he do in the evening? The SP can develop more of a sense of who the patient is if he actually imitates part of the lifestyle he imagines the patient is living.

Along these lines, let me illustrate what one 74-year-old man did to better understand the patient he was hired to portray.

The patient is an avid swimmer who was in training for an upcoming swim meet when he began to get severe pain in his right shoulder. The pain was keeping him from his daily 6 a.m. practice swim in the ocean. The patient is coming to see his doctor to get relief so that he can get back to training as soon as possible because he is preparing to defend his reigning championship in his age group during the upcoming race.

As you might imagine, the older men we had hired to play this patient had little understanding of the motivation behind this patient's passion for swimming. They wondered what kind of a "nut" this guy must be. But at the beginning of the second training session, one of the SPs had changed his tune about the patient. He was enthusiastic and full of details about the new understanding he had of the patient as a swimmer. In response to one of the other SP's comments, "You got one heck of a fantasy life, buddy!" he replied, "On the contrary—I went down to the ocean where these guys work out and spent a fair amount of time with them this week. They're in their wet suits by 5:30 in the morning ready to spend an hour or so swimming. There are a bunch of them doing this—and they all love it. They feel it's keeping them *alive*. You know, not just living—not just existing. . . ." And on and on he went.

The SP said he stopped short of getting in the water with the swimmers, although he had a real sense of their enthusiasm and the feel of the ocean setting where they spend a couple of hours every day. And he provided plenty of backstory that helped all the SPs get a feel for what had motivated this particular patient to seek the urgent medical help he felt he needed in order to keep swimming. The SP's curiosity about the patient's lifestyle changed the whole tone of the other SPs' interactions with each other and inspired some real understanding of the patient that they were preparing to portray.

You can also encourage the SPs to keep a journal of their observations while "living as the patient." They can journal for their own benefit and, if they feel comfortable enough, share their perceptions with you and the other SPs at the next session. Some of these SP journal observations have been so astute that they have been incorporated into the case materials. (Of course, any insights that become part of the training materials should be elaborations of the core intent of the case, not material that alters that core meaning.)

A Suggestion for Assisting the SPs to Remember Facts and Give Information Appropriately

If you are concerned about any of the SPs being able to remember the facts of the case, suggest that they carefully go through the case materials, writing down each of the facts on a 3×5 card. Then have them write one or several questions that might elicit that fact on the other side of the card. Any fact on the checklist that may only be given if the medical student directly asks a closed-ended question related to the answer should also be marked "May not volunteer." They can then practice remembering the facts by interviewing themselves with the questions on the cards.

Essentially, the SPs are creating flash cards containing the facts. The very nature of making and using the flash cards engages multiple senses in recalling the facts: tactile, visual, auditory. SPs of all ages who have had trouble with the facts of a case have testified to the effectiveness of this method of memorization.

Flash cards can help the SPs in another way. Often inappropriately volunteering checklist information on the part of the SPs is simply a matter of not being familiar enough with the checklist. However, volunteering could be a more involved issue if the SPs have been asked in the case materials to respond to certain kinds of open-ended questions by giving answers that may include one or two specific checklist items. The idea behind having the SP give a relevant answer to open-ended questions is to reward the medical students for their appropriate use of this important communication skill, rather than to eliminate the use of open-ended questions by always having the SPs push the students back to asking closed-ended questions.

If the issue is inappropriately volunteering checklist items, give the SPs a number of open-ended questions to put on additional flash cards to weave into their practice interviews before the next session.

You are now ready to select and review the video recordings you want to use in Training Session Two—and make all other necessary preparations for the upcoming sessions.

CHAPTER EIGHT

Training Session Two: Learning to Use the Checklist

Observing and recalling the medical student's behavior in order to accurately complete the checklist are among the most demanding tasks for all standardized patients—for the experienced and inexperienced, for the skilled actor and the non-actor alike. Nevertheless, we can help our SPs become proficient in checklist recording and improve their accuracy through the following means:

- *Giving the SPs practice in filling out the checklist—as a separate skill from performance.* There are many ways to provide the SPs with practice in filling out checklists and in reinforcing the necessity of using the guide to the checklist as a reference whenever they have a question about how to answer a given checklist item (see Appendixes A4 and A5). The method laid out in this chapter allows the SPs to experience, as a separate task, the requirements regarding checklist accuracy without yet worrying about the nuances of their own portrayal of the patient case.

- *Coaching the SPs and sharing techniques with them that research has shown enhances the correspondence between the completed checklist and what actually happened during the clinical encounter.* The accuracy of the final scores that the medical students receive on their CPX performances in part directly correlates with how successful we have been in coaching the SPs to accurately understand and interpret the checklist items, as well as to accurately observe, interpret, recall, and record the students' behavior on the checklists. (See Heine, Garman, Wallace, Bartos, & Richards,

2003, "An Analysis of Standardized Patient Checklist Errors" and the article's bibliography.) The accuracy of the students' scores also depends on how diligent we, as coaches, have been in monitoring and giving feedback to our SPs on their performances and completed checklists throughout every CPX exam administration (Wallace et al., 1999).

Principles for Checklist Coaching

Here are some general principles to follow when coaching the SPs to use the checklist.

Always Have the SPs Fill Out Each Checklist Immediately After Each Encounter

The SP has the best chance of being accurate if nothing intervenes between the clinical encounter and his recording of what happened during the encounter.

Require the SPs to Anchor Every Checklist Response to a Specific Action From the Encounter

Throughout the training, encourage the SPs to get into the habit of filling out the checklist in this manner. The specific action connected to the SP's response on a given checklist item might be something the student did or said, or it might be the SP's own action or reaction that she remembers; for example, if the SP is having trouble remembering whether or not the student palpated the lower right quadrant of her abdomen, she might be able to retrieve this memory by recalling whether or not she winced in pain during the physical exam.

This is why it is also helpful to have the SP's response built into each history item on the checklist. SPs find this particularly useful in the early stages of training when they are learning the facts of the case, first becoming acquainted with the checklists, and during the practice encounters as they are discovering what may and may not be volunteered.

If we do not encourage specific recall from the SPs, some of them will fill out the checklist by how they felt about the student. This way of operating is particularly prevalent when the SPs are having trouble recalling whether or not the student asked a specific question or did a particular physical exam maneuver that is on the checklist. If they liked the student or are uncomfortable docking him for something they cannot recall, the SPs are likely to give credit on some items that the student did not do, which creates a kind of halo effect that can produce a string of yeses on their checklist. Conversely, though less frequently, if the SPs disliked the student, they are sometimes unconsciously inclined not to give him credit for an item or items that he actually did perform.

Let the SPs Know That Checklist Accuracy Becomes More Challenging With Each Successive Student

Not surprisingly, the most common reason for checklist errors has to do with faulty recall. Checklist accuracy becomes more difficult with each new student because the events in the multiple encounters start to blend together. While filling out the checklist, the SPs begin to have difficulty remembering whether it was the student that they had just seen who had done something or asked a certain question, or whether it was a student they had seen previously.

Let the SPs Know Which Checklists Are Likely to Be the Most Difficult to Accurately Fill Out

The checklists that seem to be the most difficult are those just prior to a break and the last encounters of an exam administration. Not only do the encounters start to blend together, but fatigue sets in, which is why it is important to build a break into any exam that is longer than six stations. For instance, in an eight-station exam, it is the fourth encounter (the one before the break) and the seventh and eighth encounters that the SPs consistently report are the most challenging for them in terms of accurate recall. It is helpful for the SPs to know about this phenomenon ahead of time so that they can redouble their efforts at concentration, or use other techniques that help them work with each student "as if that encounter were the first."

A break gives both the SPs and the students a chance to relax and renew their energy. When they go back to the next segment of the exam, it is almost like starting over fresh because the break has given them separation from the students they had seen previously.

Make Sure the SPs Fill Out all of the Checklist Items Before They Write Their Comments

The way the checklist is *laid out* often determines the way it is *filled out*. One of the most common ways to design a checklist is to lay out the items in the order the student will likely proceed through the encounter. For example, the checklist might start out with history items, followed by physical examination maneuvers, then patient education or information sharing items, and finally, by items related to physician–patient interaction (PPI)/communication skills that apply to the entire encounter. This layout works well because as it happens the history taking, physical examination, and information-sharing items are the more difficult ones for the SPs to recall accurately and therefore should be the first items that the SPs fill out on the checklist.

The PPI items and the comment section should be the last items filled out on the checklist because the feelings that the SPs have about the interaction and their relationship with the student are the easiest parts of the clinical encounter to remember. On the last page of the checklist, the SPs will have a chance to give feedback in the form of written comments to the medical students on their interaction with them. At the head of this comment section is a case summary paragraph called "From the Patient's Perspective," which the SPs will become familiar with during training as a touchstone for their performances and as a trigger for the comments they write when giving feedback to the students (see Appendix A4 and the end of chapter 9 for more on feedback).

The Goal of Training Session Two

The purpose of Training Session Two is to familiarize the standardized patients with the checklist and the guide to the checklist and to give them practice in their use. By the end of this session you should feel confident that all the SPs (a) understand the intent of each checklist item and (b) can accurately record the student's behavior that they observed on the sample video recordings.

The Training Setting

This session should take place in a conference room that can accommodate the progressive interview and that also has a small conference table and a video playback unit with a screen large enough for you and all the SPs to easily see details of the recorded student doctor/SP interactions you will be watching together during this session.

Summary of the Training Activities

There are three main activities in Training Session Two. The coach needs to:

1. Do a brief progressive interview that allows the SPs to demonstrate their progress in the portrayal of the patient and gives the coach an opportunity to rectify any performance issues.

2. Answer any questions the SPs have about the guide to the checklist. This is also an opportunity for the coach to highlight and discuss any checklist items that may need further clarification.
3. Have the SPs practice filling out the checklists while watching previously recorded student/SP encounters on video.

Working With the Checklists

The SPs Will Practice Filling Out Checklists While Using the Guide to the Checklist

The checklists they will complete will be on each of three previously video-recorded student encounters of their case.

All of the SPs' Responses to the Items on the Checklist Will Be Reviewed and Compared After Each Encounter

Following their viewing of the video of each clinical encounter, the coach and the SPs should discuss the responses they have recorded on the checklist. It is at this point—particularly after the first attempt at filling out the checklist—that the SPs are often surprised to see how differently they each responded. Even if the accuracy and correspondence among the SPs is disappointing, neither you nor they should be discouraged because these differences in response will graphically demonstrate to them the need for practice in filling out the checklist and the necessity of using the guide to the checklist.

The Coach Will Lead a Discussion of Any Checklist Items About Which the SPs Disagree

There is no reason to waste energy discussing items about which there is complete agreement. By focusing the discussions only on items about which there is disagreement, the SPs learn exactly what they need to know about the specific items on the checklist that need their attention. Where there is disagreement on an item, someone has made an error. Where there is an error, someone's recall is faulty, the SP's interpretation of the intent of the item is incorrect, or the student's approach to an element in the encounter caused confusion that resulted in an incorrect interpretation of what the student did during the encounter.

All of this is exactly what you, as a coach, want to have happen. It is the very stuff that will help the SPs grow into a deeper, more refined understanding of the checklist. Each time they disagree on an item on the checklist, see it as another opportunity to encourage the SPs to use the guide to the checklist as the means to sort out the correct response to the item in question. Eventually, the SPs will become so familiar with the checklist and the guide that they will know on which page and where on the page each item is located. These items will become anchors for them as they fill out the checklist during the exam (whether on paper or on a computer).

Obtaining the Practice Videos

The following are a few of the most commonly asked questions about the videos needed for this session.

Where Do the Video Recordings for This Session Come From?

The best way to obtain videos of SP performances is from a previous year's exam. Do not pick the best or the worst student encounters because both kinds are too easy to score. It is a much greater challenge to have the SPs work with middle-of-the-road students—those who do some things well, some not so well. The SPs then have to make decisions that are similar to the kinds of challenges they will experience with most of the medical students in an actual exam.

Where Do I Get the Videos If the Case Is New and Has Not Been Used in a Previous Exam?

If you are dealing with only one or two new cases, you can do a quick training of a single SP, call in several residents or medical students who have already passed the CPX in a previous year, and record them going through the case. A secondary benefit of creating these videos is that you get a preview of aspects of the case that might require special attention during regular training.

What If all the Cases in an Exam Are New?

In chapter 11, there is information on how to handle Training Sessions Two and Three when you are faced with putting on a CPX with completely new cases or when the majority of SPs are new or inexperienced and will need more coaching of their performances for the exam. (See chapter 11, Training Options: Variations on the Training Sessions.)

Reminders

Remember to Save all the SPs' Completed Checklists

This is especially important if you want to track the progress of the SPs in terms of their accuracy. It is also hard data that the CPX advisory committee will find useful if you have to decide whether or not to replace an SP.

Letting the SPs know that you will be saving their checklists is a tangible way to indicate that you care about their accuracy and improvement. When you tell them this, also inform them that saving their checklists is part of standard operating procedure, not a threat of dismissal. Continuing to maintain an atmosphere of encouragement in which the SPs know that you are confident in their ability will give them the motivation to succeed according to the standards you have set.

Caveat: Set your standards high, but not too high. Remember, there are still several training sessions to go. If the SPs are not 100% accurate in filling out the checklists but you are confident that they understand the intent behind each of the items, if they are eagerly looking up information in the guide whenever they are not sure how to fill out an item, and if they are sharp observers of student behavior and are at least 80% accurate— do not worry. Their checklist skills will improve with practice during the next training sessions.

However, if there are any SPs who are having unusual difficulty in accurately completing the checklists, you will need to decide whether additional training might help or whether to let the SP go (and proceed with training without a backup SP for the case).

Session Two Training Activities (Estimated Time: 3 Hours)

Do a Brief, Focused Progressive Interview

Because the emphasis of this session is on checklist accuracy, unless you build in a progressive interview, you will have no sense of whether or not the SPs are improving in their portrayal of the case. First, check to see if the SPs have any questions on the training materials. Then, do a brief progressive interview of no more than 20 minutes, which concentrates on performance issues that concern you most. This should be enough to give you either the reassurance that all is going well on the performance level or the confidence to consider further coaching or dismissal of an SP who has not improved. This performance "check-in" also gives the SPs a sense of the issues they still need to work on for the next session.

Elicit Questions From the SPs About the Guide to the Checklist

The substance of the guide to the checklist consists of an explanation of the intent of each item, where needed, and examples of the kinds of student questions or actions that merit credit. Certain items, if warranted, may include specific examples of what does *not* merit credit (see Appendix A5, Guide to the Checklist).

First, check to see if the SPs have any questions that might have arisen from their review of the guide to the checklist, which they did in preparation for this session. Besides answering their questions, you might want to point out specific kinds of circumstances that you know can cause confusion. For example:

> Let's say one of the checklist items reads, "The student asked if I have ever had cancer." But what if, instead of asking the question the way it is stated in the checklist, a student asks something like, "Do you have any medical problems?" or "Have you been pretty healthy?" If the patient is healthy and has not had cancer and the SP responds correctly to the student's question with "Yes, I have been pretty healthy," does the SP give the student credit (on the checklist item "asked-if-I've-ever-had-cancer") for having found this information out indirectly?

Herein lies the dilemma. Sometimes certain aspects of a case are not as straightforward as they seem to be, no matter how diligently we have tried to clarify the training materials and the checklist. When medical students ask open-ended questions of this sort, we do not know what is on their minds. Therefore, if the designers of the checklist want to know specifically if the student is thinking about cancer, we need to make sure that the SPs know how to deal with these kinds of open-ended questions when they are asked. (For more details on this topic, see PPI/Communication Skills in chapter 2, Clinical Skills: Acquiring the Basic Doctoring Skills.)

Introduce the SPs to How to Fill Out the Checklist (Using the Computer, Other Electronic Protocols, or Scantron Bubbling)

In order not to complicate the goals of this session, I encourage using printed copies of the actual checklists that the SPs will be using during the exam. If the SPs will use a computer or any other electronic technology to record the student's behavior during the exam, you can introduce the procedures for recording their responses electronically during this session, but postpone the actual use of the electronic devices until the SPs are well grounded in their understanding of the meaning of the checklist items. By the next training session the SPs should be ready to incorporate the use of this technology.

Show Videos of Three Different Students Interviewing SPs Portraying Their Case

This is the heart of the practical experience for this session. While watching the videos, do not avoid answering questions that arise regarding the portrayals of the SPs, but keep in mind that the focus of the SPs should be on the medical student—what she says, what she does—for the purpose of learning how to accurately fill out the checklist. The following guidelines for *when* the SPs should fill out their checklists during this session are designed to help the SPs progress in their familiarity with, and skill in, completing the checklist.

When Watching the First Two Videos, the SPs Will Fill Out Checklists <u>While</u> They Are Watching the Encounter

This process focuses the SPs on *observation,* giving them two complete encounters to understand the checklist items themselves, before also having to worry about remembering what the student did after the encounter is finished.

Caveat: When filling out a checklist as the encounter is unfolding on the video, the SPs may sometimes miss a checklist item because they look away from the screen to mark a previous item they had observed. This potential occasion-for-error is important for the coach and the SPs to understand, because an error of omission is one of the reasons that the SPs' checklists might differ during this training session. This is also true during an exam when you compare checklists for accuracy—comparing yours, which you filled out *during* the encounter, with theirs, which they will have filled out *after* the encounter.

Even if you have already made "keys" to the checklist ahead of time for the videos you have selected, you might want to fill out another checklist while each video is playing during the session. If there are differences between your keys and the checklists you fill out during the session, the discrepancies can be a clue to the potential difficulty of certain items. However, be aware that such discrepancies can also simply mean that you were distracted while filling out one of the checklists.

While Watching the Third Video, the SPs Will Fill Out the Checklist <u>By Recall</u> After the Encounter is Over—Taking as Long as Needed

SPs are usually surprised at how different it feels to fill out the checklist *after* the encounter. But by the time they have completed this exercise, they should have a much better sense of what will be involved when they have to fill out checklists following their own performance of the case.

Many SPs worry about being able to complete the checklist in the time allotted. If you sense this concern among your SPs, you can offer to time their completion of this last checklist so that they can see how close they come to finishing within the exam timeframe. Be sure to let anyone who does not finish on time know that speed will come with practice.

Give the SPs as much extra time as they need to complete the checklist during this session. Make sure that everyone understands that this session is about clarity of understanding and accuracy, not about speed.

After Viewing Each Video, the Coach and the SPs Will Compare Checklists for Uniformity of Response

Reviewing and comparing checklists should reveal any problems that exist

- for the SPs in filling out the checklist.
- with the guide to the checklist.
- with the checklist itself.

When the completed checklists are compared, invariably it becomes clear that certain items carry different interpretations for the SPs. There is no better way to bring the coaches and the SPs together in their understanding than by comparing incongruent responses and figuring out why each person marked the item the way they did. These discussions are also helpful in determining which SPs could have potential problems with checklist accuracy and in which areas those SPs might require extra help.

In addition, the outcome of these checklist-comparison discussions consistently brings to light items that might warrant changes, additions, or clarifications to the guide and/or the checklist.

Guidelines for Leading the Training Discussions During the Checklist Comparison

Discuss Only the Checklist Items Where There Are Discrepancies in the SPs' Responses, or There Are Outright Errors

What you are concerned about in the review of checklists is finding out where there are misunderstandings, misperceptions, or faulty judgments. As mentioned earlier, the most efficient means to accomplish this task is to focus on items where there is disagreement—or on any item where all the SPs' responses are in agreement, but they are all wrong!

Have the SPs identify each error on their checklist by highlighting it with a marker. Do not allow them to erase and correct their errors. By highlighting their mistakes, it makes it easy for the SPs to get an overview of their errors on each checklist. It also makes it easier for you to identify errors and SPs who are having trouble with accuracy.

Be sure you highlight your own checklist errors as well. Doing this lets the SPs know that you are willing to follow the same rules you set for them. This is especially important during this session because SPs sometimes become discouraged—even at this early stage—if they are not 100% accurate on all of their checklists.

Determine if the Discrepancies in Item Responses Are a Matter of Recall

Research has shown that when SPs err in recording the student's behavior, they usually err *in favor* of the student (Heine, 2003). Often when SPs are not sure if a student performed a given item, they tend to give the student the benefit of the doubt, or they fall back on how they felt in general about the encounter. Therefore, asking each SP to identify what the student actually did in the encounter that warranted their positive response on the checklist is good practice. By encouraging the SPs, from the very beginning, to anchor their responses to actual recalled behaviors, you are helping them to develop the habit of filling out the checklist item by item, not by their overall feeling toward the student.

Consider Reviewing the Video to Resolve any Recall Discrepancies in the SPs' Checklist Responses

If the SPs are split between a positive and a negative response and the discussions get bogged down because you have no pertinent annotations on your checklist key, it might be necessary to review the video of the encounter to resolve the discrepancy. But remember that finding the section on the video that relates to a given item can take precious time away from the actual practice of filling out the checklists. So use your judgment regarding the value or necessity of such a review.

Identify Whether Everyone Understands the Item in the Same Way

As obvious as this seems, asking the SPs upfront to share their interpretation of an item under discussion can save a good deal of training time.

Preparation of the SPs for Training Session Three

Explain That Training Session Three Will Focus on Combining Performance With Checklist Accuracy

By the end of the next session, the SPs should have practiced the simulation enough so that they are ready to realistically and accurately perform the case. They should know the facts and be able to perform the simulated physical findings as if they were second nature to them (and not have to think about the right answer or response in the midst of their performances).

In addition, the SPs, for the first time, will be filling out checklists *after their own performances*. They should prepare for this by carefully reviewing the checklist and the guide to the checklist prior to the next session.

Remind the SPs to Bring Their Calendars to the Next Session

The SPs will set their performance schedule by signing up for specific CPX exam administrations at the end of Training Session Three.

The Coach's Preparation for Training Session Three

Consider Making a Cheat Sheet

If you will be the only coach working with the SPs during the next session, and particularly if you are a new coach, consider making a cheat sheet as support for the next session's interviews. A cheat sheet is a list of all the possible questions you, as the coach, might want to ask the SPs during the next session's practice encounters. If you are a new coach, the next session can be challenging because you will be handling many tasks simultaneously: interviewing, observing, and coaching the SPs in their performances, as well as having the last word on the accuracy of their checklists. A cheat sheet can give you the confidence to work with the SPs in a more relaxed way so that you are not totally absorbed as the interviewer (in the role of the medical student). The cheat sheet allows you to focus more of your attention on the SPs' performances and on coaching them when needed.

Do Not Create a Cheat Sheet From the Checklist Alone

The best way to put the cheat sheet together is to go through both the checklist *and* the training materials to create questions that will elicit specific patient information. Be sure also to include questions about the patient that are *not* on the checklist or in the training materials—for example, questions about related medical problems that the patient does not have. This will give the SPs a thorough and more realistic practice session than if the cheat sheet simply follows what is contained on the checklist. During the CPX, the medical students will ask all kinds of questions, some of which may not relate to what is in the training materials, so practicing in the same manner is the best way to prepare the standardized patients for what they are going to experience.

If you are not a clinician and are having trouble coming up with questions that are not in the training materials, it is reasonable to consider asking a faculty clinician to help you with ideas for questions a student would be likely to ask such a patient.

Combine Both Closed-Ended and Open-Ended Questions

When and how information related to the checklist items is to be revealed by the SPs to the students needs to be crystal clear in the training materials. Most checklist items are not to be revealed unless the student specifically asks closed-ended questions. However, there are times when the faculty want to reward the medical student by allowing the SPs to give certain information (which may include a specific checklist item) when the student asks an appropriate open-ended question. This is the kind of information that must be carefully described in the training materials so that the SPs understand what is being asked of them (see last page of Appendix A3). Coaches must give the SPs plenty of practice in making these kinds of decisions during the training sessions. When an SP makes an error by inappropriately volunteering a checklist item in training, it is the best way for all the SPs to learn what circumstances trap them into volunteering information. The actual experience of volunteering a checklist item (or in noticing when someone else gets caught doing so) is powerful—more powerful than anything you can tell them in words. (See chapter 2 for more details on using open-ended questions.)

Schedule a Second Coach or Assistant to Work With You During the Next Session

Training Session Three is one of the most intense sessions you will conduct during the SPs' training. Therefore, if you schedule someone else—another coach, a nurse, a physician's assistant, or a medical student (who is in a class ahead of the students designated to take the CPX)—to interview the SPs in your place during the next session, it will free you up to observe the whole process from a more objective point of view. You can then watch the encounters and coach the SPs on their portrayals after each encounter, fill out checklists during the encounters, make notes on how the checklist items were handled by the interviewer, and so on. In short, having an assistant do some or all of the interviewing will make your job as a coach much more manageable during this critical session when everything will be coming together for the first time.

The Coach's Preparation for Training Session Four, the Practice Exam, and the CPX

Training Session Four

If you do not already have the requisite number of acceptances, continue recruitment of a clinician for each case to validate the authenticity of the SPs' portrayals.

The Practice Exam and the CPX

Continue recruitment if you still need residents to participate as examinees during the Practice Exam.

Confer with the administrator responsible for the exam logistics to make sure that all of your needs and the needs of the SPs are being integrated into the logistical plans for conducting the Practice Exam and the CPX. Someone other than the SP coach needs to be responsible for the logistics of the Practice Exam and all administrations of the CPX. This is important so that you can concentrate on monitoring and giving feedback to your SPs on their performances and checklists throughout each and every exam administration, in order to maintain the high level of accuracy the SPs have attained during training. Therefore, anything to do with proctoring, timing, recording video—or any other administrative responsibilities required to run the CPX—should be handled by someone else who is specifically designated to coordinate the critical logistical details that are so important to a well-orchestrated performance examination.

CHAPTER NINE

Training Session Three: Putting It All Together (Performance, Checklist, Feedback)

During the first two training sessions, the SPs had an opportunity to try on the role of the patient by performing parts of the case in two different progressive interviews as well as separate practice in filling out the checklist and using the guide to the checklist. In this third training session, the SPs will have a chance to put these performance and checklist activities together for the first time. In addition, the SPs will learn one other skill: how to give feedback from the patient's perspective by writing comments about their interaction with the medical student immediately following the clinical encounter. These written comments compose the final segment on the last page of the checklist (see Appendix A4). When the SPs are well trained to provide this feedback, both students and faculty find these individualized written comments from the SPs an insightful adjunct to the statistical reports on the students' clinical communication skills, which are derived from the ratings the SPs give on the Patient–Physician Interaction items.

Because this is a key session requiring us, as coaches, to provide the SPs with practice on the multiple aspects of their job as patients, this training session will take longer than any of the others. In fact, some SP coaches choose to divide this session into two training sessions to give the SPs ample practice time, or alternatively to make feedback training an altogether separate session (see chapter 11, Training Options). The complexity of the case and the experience and age of the SPs are usually the factors that help determine whether or not to create separate sessions.

However, in this chapter, I describe in detail how to put together all the portrayal, performance, checklist, and feedback elements in one session. That being the case, the emphasis in Training Session Three is on three areas that are described in detail in the material that follows: attaining authenticity and standardization of the patient's affect, achieving the highest levels of accuracy in performance of case content and checklist recording, and learning how to give effective feedback.

The Three Areas of Training Emphasis: Performance, Checklist, Feedback

Attaining Authenticity and Standardization of the Patient's Affect

The refinement of the realism, accuracy, and standardization of the emotional and psychological aspects of the SPs' patient portrayals, both during the interview and when producing the physical findings during the physical examination, initially takes place during this session (and continues through the next session and the Practice Exam). This work is critical so that the students' true competence—in dealing not only with the medical aspects but with all of the aspects of the patient's condition—can be accurately assessed. The progressive interviews in the first two training sessions gave the SPs a chance to experience performing as the patient while interpreting the case parameters in the way that each SP individually and collectively understood them. It also gave you a chance, as the coach, to adjust the SPs' performances in key areas of their portrayal during the history and information-sharing portions of the encounter. Now, in this session, you and the SPs (who from this point on will be performing full encounters individually) will refine details and perfect performances—including the physical exam findings—bringing everyone closer together in their interpretations and in how they present the challenges of the case to the students. Of course, all of this must be done under your guidance and coaching as the SPs practice reacting to whatever you or your assistant are doing as you portray a variety of student styles during the practice encounters.

Achieving the Highest Levels of Accuracy in Performance of Case Content and Checklist Recording

Although it is possible to achieve 100% factual accuracy virtually all of the time in performance, it is not humanly possible for the SPs to achieve the same perfection on the checklists. A number of studies have looked at the level of SP factual accuracy and the consistency of their performances. (If you are interested in getting a taste of the research that has been done in this area, see Petrusa, 2002; Tamblyn et al., 1997; Tamblyn, Klass, Schnabl, & Kopelow, 1991).

Although it is equally clear from the literature that SPs can be trained to a high degree of checklist accuracy, at the same time it is also clear that, for a number of reasons, it is difficult for SPs to be consistently 100% accurate in their checklist recording. Two of the factors that we know affect the SPs' checklist accuracy have to do with the quality and consistency of the training methods and the type and quality of the checklists themselves (Huber, Baroffio et al., 2005; De Champlain, Margolis, King, & Klass, 1997). Therefore, knowing this, what we can realistically expect of well-selected SPs is that they strive for 100% accuracy, but not fall below an overall accuracy rate of 85% (see bibliography in Heine et al., 2003). It is good to know that this completely attainable SP accuracy rate (and the overall accuracy rate of 95% reported by Heine in her research) is higher than the 80% rate that is "about as accurate as physicians [are] in evaluating and recording clinical performance" (Colliver & Williams, 1993, p. 455; see also Vu & Barrows, 1994). Something else we know is that when SPs make checklist errors, in the aggregate, the majority of the errors usually end up in favor of the student (Heine et al., 2003; Vu et al., 1992). (For a list of other factors, see chapter 12, p. 253. Other Measures to Ensure Consistently High SP Accuracy.)

By way of review, here is a summary of some of the key concepts we have touched on earlier in the book that will come into play during this practice session.

Performance Accuracy

Even though well-chosen standardized patients can be consistently accurate in their portrayals, there are some performance issues that can cause problems for even the best SPs. You already know that accurately memorizing and reporting the facts of a case, which remain consistent no matter who is interacting with the SP, is a relatively easy, basic task that every SP should be expected to demonstrate. Therefore, when errors are made in performance, they usually have less to do with memorization and reporting than with a number of other factors, some of the more important of which are described in the following.

- *Determining <u>when</u> it is appropriate for the SP to give information to the student.* This is especially true when the information to be given is part of the checklist. Most performance errors occur because an SP inappropriately volunteers or withholds information that is on the checklist. Therefore, to improve accuracy in performance, the meaning and import behind each checklist item must be thoroughly understood by the SPs so that they have the wherewithal to determine whether or not to give information to the medical student as the encounter unfolds. The checklist and the guide to the checklist are not instruments to be used solely for learning how to accurately record student behavior. The SPs must also regard the checklist and the guide as containing information that is integral to the accuracy of their performances.

- *Dealing appropriately with open-ended questions when the potential answers are on the checklist.* In the past, much emphasis has been placed on requiring SPs to answer checklist items *only if specifically asked.* In a sense, this requirement trains medical students in the long run to ask only closed-ended questions because they are not rewarded with information (in the same way that they are by real patients) when asking open-ended questions of the SPs during an exam. This is an outcome none of us wishes to promulgate. Consequently, SPs are now being trained to give reasonable answers (which might include a checklist item or two) for suitably asked open-ended questions. However, the SPs must be given norms for determining how to deal with such questions. Those norms must be spelled out in the training materials or the guide to the checklist so that the SPs understand the parameters for their responses. What follows is an example of a situation calling for this kind of consideration. (For other examples, see Appendix A3, Training Materials.)

> After coughing up blood for a couple of days, a patient makes an appointment to see her doctor. The earliest appointment she could get was for 2 weeks later. She has not coughed up blood in the intervening time. She tells the doctor the reason for her visit is "a cough I've had for a while that won't go away."
>
> If, after asking a series of questions pertinent to the cough, a student were to ask this patient, "Is anything else bothering you?" or "Do you have any other concerns?" or "Do you have any other symptoms?" it not only seems inappropriate, but false to have the patient respond, "No" or "What do you mean?" simply because we do not want the SP to "volunteer" the checklist item that reads, "The student asked me if I had seen blood in my sputum."
>
> This particular patient does not let the doctor know at the beginning of the encounter that she has seen blood in her sputum because she is afraid of what it might mean. But if the student doctor were to ask her any of these open-ended questions (as the case author asked the real patient), the way the patient responds belies her underlying fear, "Yes, sometimes I do see some red streaks in what I cough up, but it's not all the time." In such situations, this kind of response is appropriate, logical, and reasonable.

No matter how expertly open-ended questions are described in the case materials, as with all performance issues, a written description is not enough to ensure that the SPs have a clear enough understanding of how to consistently and accurately respond to these kinds of questions. The important concept here is that unless the SPs have a variety of opportunities to practice and are specifically coached in how to handle open-ended questions, they will unavoidably make errors. Therefore, during this training session and the next, *it is imperative that the interviewer ask open-ended questions repeatedly throughout the encounters* and give the SPs a diversity of experiences and challenges in this area.

- *Coping effectively with the consequences of case familiarity and fatigue.*

  After the SPs have performed a case a number of times, they can become so familiar with the portrayal that they sometimes, without realizing it, begin to improvise information that can be detrimental to the case. In addition, after having worked with a number of students in a given administration, fatigue sets in and one encounter begins to blend with another. You may see the latter phenomenon during this third training session. The SPs must learn to let go of the previous encounter and renew their concentration before working with each student, each time they perform. The ability to let go, concentrate, and approach each encounter as if it were the first is not only important in maintaining accuracy and authenticity in the standardized patients' performances but is also a key factor in assuring the accuracy of the SPs' checklists.

Checklist Accuracy

Because it is possible for the SPs to produce checklists that are at times completely free of error, it is wise for us to routinely set the bar high for them, without being unreasonable about our expectations. Conversely, if any SP consistently has more than a 15% overall error rate on the checklists during this session, a decision is in order. You should know by the end of this session which SPs will be able to perform at the level required—and which will not.

You may ask, why is it possible for SPs to attain 100% accuracy more consistently in their performance of a case than it is for them to fill out the checklists with the same accuracy? The reason for this discrepancy is partially in the nature of the two activities themselves. Performance happens in the moment; checklist recording happens on recall. It is easier to respond correctly in the moment than it is to remember exactly what happened after the encounter for two reasons: first, the SP is required to mentally note and remember what the student is doing at the same time that she herself is performing in the encounter; and second, because it becomes progressively more difficult to keep track of what happened in each successive encounter after seeing several students in a row.

However, as mentioned earlier, it *is* possible for SPs to achieve a consistently high level of accuracy in checklist recording, even though they cannot be expected to be 100% accurate all of the time. In fact, no one can be expected to be 100% accurate in checklist recording all of the time, including observers who might be watching the interactions of the encounters from a monitoring room and filling out checklists simultaneously. We cannot be absolutely sure that the checklist of the person filling in the responses *during* the encounter is any more accurate than the checklist of the SP who fills in responses *following* the encounter. This is especially true regarding items that are scored "Not Done," due to the fact that the observer–recordist might have missed something in the encounter because of a wandering mind or because of distractions in the monitoring room or wherever the checklist is being filled out. The only time one can reasonably be assured that the observer–recordist is correct (and the SP *incorrect* on a given item) is if the observer has written a note on the checklist about what she observed the student actually say or do.

Learning How to Give Effective Feedback

The new area for the SPs to learn during this session has to do with how to give thoughtful, supportive, and beneficial written feedback to the students on their clinical performances. (This information is covered in detail later in this chapter under Training the SPs to Give Effective Written Feedback.)

The Goal of Training Session Three

The purpose of Training Session Three is to assist the standardized patients in combining several skill sets. The SPs' portrayals must be realistic; their facts accurate, timely, and pertinent; and the challenges to the students appropriate for the clinical encounter. Simultaneously, the SP coach must exercise the SPs' abilities to observe, recall, and accurately fill out the checklist. Finally, the SPs must learn how to give (and practice writing) effective, individualized feedback to the medical student from the point of view of the patient the SPs are portraying.

The Training Setting

This session requires a large examination room to accommodate you, your assistant (if you have one), and all the SPs. The performing SP and your assistant (or you) who will be playing the part of the medical student will be working on and around the exam table. The observing SPs (and you whenever the assistant is doing the interviewing) will be sitting in a single line of chairs positioned in the exam room for optimal viewing of the activities in the practice encounters. The observing SPs should be encouraged to get up and move around during the physical examination so that they can see exactly what the interviewer (playing the role of the medical student) is doing. The performing SP and the interviewer simply proceed as if the others are not in the room.

Summary of the Training Activities

These are the primary activities to accomplish in this session:

- The coach will teach the SPs how to give written feedback to the students.
- Each SP will go through at least two complete practice encounters with the coach or the coach's assistant in the role of the medical student.
- All SPs will fill out checklists on each encounter and practice writing comments about the encounter from the perspective of the patient they are portraying.
- The coach will teach the SPs how to fill out the checklists on the particular electronic data collection system that the SPs will be using during the CPX. From now on, all of the checklists the SPs fill out when *performing* the case should be done on a computer. The observing SPs can continue to fill out printed versions of the electronic checklist.

Reminders

Use an Additional Coach or Clinician as an Assistant in This Session

You should have scheduled an additional coach or clinician—a nurse practitioner, a physician's assistant, or a primary care clinician—to assist you during this session. The advantage of having an assistant interview the patients, in lieu of yourself, is twofold:

- A different interviewer gives the SPs a chance to work with someone other than yourself—with someone who has a different style and way of approaching the patient; in essence, a little sample of the variety they will experience when working with the students during the CPX.
- An assistant can provide you the opportunity to step back from direct immersion in the practice encounters, allowing you to observe, coach, and take notes on how events unfolded in the encounters. In short, having someone else assume the role of the medical student with the patients allows you to focus on the overall picture and to gain a more objective view of how the integration of skills is proceeding for the SPs.

Use These Suggested Protocols for the Practicing of Filling Out Checklists in This Session

- Because they will be performing the encounter, the person portraying the medical student (the coach, the assisting coach or clinician) and the performing SP must fill out their checklists *after* the encounter.
- As a warm-up, the observers will fill out their checklists *during* the first round of practice encounters for each SP.
- On all subsequent practice encounters, *everyone* will fill out checklists *after* the encounter.

Time Each of the Practice Encounters, Including Completion of the Checklist and the Writing of Comments, Using the Exam Timeframe

Using the exam timeframe as a guideline will help focus the encounters, allowing each SP to experience at least two complete practice encounters of different interviewing styles. It will also give the SPs a feel for how long each exam encounter will last and how much time they will actually have to complete their checklists and comments.

Have all the SPs Fill Out Checklists Under the Same Circumstances as in an Exam

In other words, during this training session, Session Four, and the Practice Exam, the SPs should be practicing with the very checklists that they will be filling out during the CPX. For example, if scannable checklists are to be used, then everyone should be using checklists in that format. If the data are to be collected electronically, it is equally important that the SPs practice from now on using the computers that they will use during the actual CPX so that the equipment and format become second nature to them.

Record All of the Encounters

Consider video recording all of the encounters during this session for reference purposes. It can also be helpful to review these videos with an individual SP if you decide that additional training is necessary.

Save All of the Checklists

Along with the video recordings, the SPs' checklists can be used as data to confirm their progress, or lack of progress if dismissal becomes necessary.

Use a Cheat Sheet to Improve the Effectiveness of the Practice Encounters

If you do not have an assistant working with you during this session (and are new to training), use the cheat sheet that you created for this session— a list of all the questions you can think of asking the SP, including all the checklist items—to jog your memory before each practice encounter. Remember, however, that the use of a cheat sheet is primarily an aid to assist new SP coaches. So, if you are an experienced SP coach, you likely will no longer need such a prompting device.

As you interview the patient, do not slavishly read the questions one after another in the order you have written them down—unless, of course, you intend to give the SP practice interacting with a student who buries his head in his clipboard, taking voluminous notes. Worse yet, do not merely read down the list of questions on the checklist. This will ultimately do more damage than good because the SPs will start to anticipate encounters happening in a fixed fashion. Mix and match the questions with each practice encounter. Otherwise, the SPs will not be prepared for the fact that no encounter is ever like any other.

The best way to use the cheat sheet is to review it just before doing a practice encounter with the idea of formulating a plan of action. For instance, you might decide to perform certain parts of the physical exam correctly, others incorrectly, and leave out yet other parts entirely. You might decide to do the same thing with the history. Or you might choose to follow one line of questioning, sticking to it no matter what the patient tells you. This kind of variety gives the SPs practice in responding to different types of students and in writing comments about how particular medical students' styles of interviewing affected the patient.

If you have created your own cheat sheet, reviewing it in this manner will remind you of all the things you researched and thought about while creating it. Once you have reviewed it, take a few notes on your clipboard about what you want to do, put the cheat sheet aside, and do the interview!

You'll be surprised at how confident you are and, after a short time, how instinctive your interviewing becomes—ultimately making the cheat sheet unnecessary.

Give the SPs Practice in Responding to Different Styles and Approaches to the Interview

Here is the opportunity for you or your assistant to get into the act by taking on different roles. By portraying different types of medical students—confident, distracted, shy, distant, friendly, intense, and so on— you help prepare the SPs to interact with any kind of student they might encounter no matter how varied the approach. Cultivating different student styles/approaches might take some time, but the more you observe students working with patients, the better you will become at imitating the students' styles. You can learn how to do this from direct observation or from watching videos of actual student encounters with SPs performing any kind of case.

The idea behind portraying different styles and approaches to the interview is to prepare the SPs for *any* circumstance they might encounter. Having learned the framework of the case and the guidelines for revealing key information, playing the interview in different ways allows the SPs to practice realistically improvising the interaction (developing authenticity), and at the same time, staying within the case guidelines (ensuring standardization).

For certain types of cases, it is *essential* to portray different types of medical students during practice. These are the types of cases in which the SP's response depends on the student's attitude and manner of dealing with the patient—cases in which the patient's portrayal is determined by the student's interaction style and communication skills. Here is an example of what I mean.

> Brittany Eisler, the adolescent patient we met in an earlier chapter, has been brought to the clinic for a check-up because she's been getting short of breath when she does any kind of exercise. Other than this exercise-induced asthma, Brittany has no other medical problems, but she is drinking some alcohol with her boyfriend. She is on the pill, but her boyfriend very irregularly uses condoms. Her parents know nothing about her substance use or that she is sexually active. The way the medical student approaches Brittany and whether he is able to build trust are key to how this teenager will respond, to how much information she will give, and whether or not she will be honest about what is going on in her life.
>
> If the student demands information from the patient, or lectures her, or treats her like a child and is condescending, he will get different

information than the student who establishes rapport with Brittany by any of the following means: letting her know that what goes on between the two of them is confidential, praising her for using birth control to protect herself from getting pregnant, finding out if she is worried about getting a sexually transmitted disease, exploring why she hasn't asked her boyfriend to use condoms (rather than lecturing her on this subject), validating how difficult her situation is, and then reassuring her that his concerns as the student doctor are similar to hers, leading to an exploration of options for how she might initiate a conversation with her boyfriend about condom use.

Take the Training Seriously, But Have a Good Time

If, from their practice experiences, your SPs are growing in their understanding of the patient, improving in their performance of the case as well as in accuracy on the checklists, and, at the same time, you are all having a laugh or two and learning a little more about what it means to be human from the patient's circumstances, you know you have created the right environment for training. Training should be both intense and fun.

Remember That This Training Session Is Still a Screening for Your SPs

Training decisions can also sometimes be difficult decisions. If there are insurmountable problems with any SP, now is the time to either replace or eliminate him from the roster and work with the remaining SPs. Waiting any longer will not improve the situation and will probably only make it worse. So dig in, make the hard decision, and move on.

Before Starting the Practice Encounters, Train the SPs to Give Effective Written Feedback

Obtaining SP feedback on the students' communication skills is important because it supports the students' growing awareness of how their behaviors are affecting their interactions with their patients. No one can do this as effectively as SPs who are well trained, skillful, objective, and empathic in giving feedback. In fact, the SPs' feedback on the medical students' communication skills is one of the noteworthy and unique contributions that the SPs make to the students' learning.

Although you might not currently require your SPs to give individualized written feedback on high-stakes clinical skills examinations, I encourage you to consider doing so for several reasons. The individualized comments that the SPs give from the patient's perspective mean so much more—to the students who receive them, to the faculty who might have to remediate them on their PPI skills, and to the administration who might need something more personalized and descriptive to track a student's progress—than the statistical analysis of the student's performance on the PPI items alone can give.

Therefore, I have included a separate discussion of the importance of this kind of feedback from the SPs, along with guidelines and practical suggestions on how to train them to give this individualized written feedback to the medical students. (See Training the SPs to Give Effective Written Feedback later in this chapter.)

Go Over Administrative Details

Practice Protocols That Are Part of Your Particular Data Collection System

Demonstrate and allow the SPs to go through the actual procedures they will be using during the CPX. Throughout the rest of the training, the SPs should be practicing these protocols so that they become second nature by the time the exam begins.

If the data are to be collected on paper, each checklist will need both student and standardized patient identification. Starting with this training session, have the SPs practice using whatever means you have chosen to identify each checklist. They can place all of their own labels on the checklists prior to an exam, but must place the student's ID label (their "business card") on each checklist just prior to filling it out. This system of having the students, at the end of each encounter, give the SPs a business card—which can also be a label that the SPs put on the checklist just prior to filling it out—assures that the checklist the SP is filling out is the right one for the student they have just seen.

Remind the SPs That They Will Be Practicing Verbally "Slating the Video"
(if You Do Not Have a Video System That Automatically Marks and
Identifies the Student)

Digital video and some other video recording systems automatically identify the student's name for easy retrieval, but if you do not have this technical capability, you will want the SPs to read the name and/or identification number of the student (who has just completed the encounter) into the camera so that this information is recorded on the video. This procedure ensures that the video is correctly identified and that the checklist the SP will be filling out (using the business card/label just received from the student) matches the recorded performance. This verbal slate is helpful in verifying the student's video should the written identification on the DVD be damaged or mislabeled. Reviewing a student's video-recorded encounter might be necessary if a checklist is lost for any reason or if there is a question about the student's checklist score.

Remind the SPs That They Are Not to Make Editorial Comments or Gestures at the End of Any Encounter

Sometimes SPs are tempted to make remarks or gestures in response to the encounter as soon as the medical student leaves the room. This usually happens when a student's performance is either outstanding or particularly bad. Therefore, remind the SPs not to make any visible or verbal responses or comments at any time after the encounter because they might be inadvertently recorded. The student and/or faculty might then see the SPs' reactions should the video be reviewed later. Instead, encourage the SPs to maintain their professionalism by keeping their reactions to themselves, reading the student's name and/or ID number straightforward into the camera if required, and immediately turning to the task of filling out the checklist.

Show the SPs How to Set Up and Maintain Their Exam Rooms

Once the exam room is set up for the day's administration, the SP can be the one responsible for maintaining it between encounters with the students, making sure that all exam equipment, supplies, and the student folders with findings or lab results are back in place. They can also see to it that their exam table, pillow, and the draping sheet are neatly arranged before the entrance of the next student for the following encounter.

Session Three Training Activities (Estimated Time: 3.5 Hours)

The order and timing of all activities described in this section are designed to build toward the second round of practice encounters when all the SPs will be working in the exam timeframe for performance, checklist recording, and writing comments from the patient's perspective. During this session, you, an assistant coach or a health care professional, will be practicing two complete encounters with each SP.

Performance of Two Complete, Timed Practice Encounters With Each SP

Practice Each of the Encounters in the Same Timeframe as the Actual Exam

The typical exam encounter runs 15 to 20 minutes; the typical post-encounter write-up that the students do while the SPs are filling out their checklists runs about 10 minutes. Timing the practice encounters will help the SPs get a sense of how much the students will be able to accomplish during the encounters with them and how well they themselves are doing at completing the checklists and written comments within the allotted time. During the first round of encounters, you can be more lenient about the SPs finishing on time; however, during the second round everyone needs to be able to complete all tasks within the exam timeframe.

Ask all _Observing_ SPs to Take Notes During Each Interaction

The notes the observing SPs make should be on anything that appears to be (a) factually incorrect or (b) different from their interpretation of the patient. Having the observing SPs take notes during each encounter serves several purposes:

- It keeps all SP observers actively engaged in each encounter.
- In postencounter discussions, the SPs' notes help contribute to a common understanding and interpretation of the patient.
- It is especially helpful if you happen to be the sole coach during this session because the SPs' notetaking allows you to concentrate on the interview and on the performing SP's portrayal. The observing SPs can help keep track of all the factual errors the performing SP might make. Their notes can also help you remember _which items_ on the checklist you brought up in the encounter and _how_ you brought them up.

All Coaches and SPs Will Fill Out and Review Checklists, Comments, and the SP Observation Notes After Each Practice Encounter

By having everyone do this, you will be able to identify problem areas early and can continue to work on them throughout the session. Have each SP share her written comments with the group but, as in Training Session Two, only discuss checklist items where there are discrepancies in responses. There should be no reason that you cannot resolve discrepancies, especially if a second trainer or you are filling out checklists simultaneously with the encounters. Even without the backup of an assistant or another health care professional to do the interviewing, your SPs' notetaking on the encounter should provide you with the objective data you need to determine the correct response on each of the checklist items.

Caveat: Do _not_ have the visiting health care professional fill out checklists as your backup. Because this person will not have been trained to understand the checklist items as interpreted in the guide to the checklist, her incorrect responses could confuse the SPs and take up your valuable training time explaining them to her, rather than using that time to help the *SPs* clarify their work with the checklist. The focus of this activity should be on the SPs' checklist errors, not on the health care professional's errors. Therefore, it is best to direct the assisting professional's efforts toward working directly with the SPs by doing the interviews, freeing you to observe, coach, and fill out checklists.

Suggested Focus During Each Round of the Practice Encounters

The coach(es) and/or assisting health care professional will focus on doing two rounds of encounters with the SPs in this session. The SPs' practice should focus equally on all the major activities during both rounds: performance, checklist, and writing feedback. After each practice encounter, the coach will adjust the performing SP's portrayal if necessary, elicit the notes the observing SPs wrote while watching the encounter, lead the checklist comparison and discussion among all the SPs, and give feedback after each SP reads out loud the comments they wrote on how they, as the patient, felt about the interaction skills of the student you or your assistant were portraying.

The First Round of Encounters

During the first round of encounters, your primary focus should be on the authenticity and accuracy of each SP's portrayal. Time the encounters and checklist recording, but within reason, allow everyone as much time as they need to complete all the activities, including the writing of comments at the end of the checklist.

Portrayal. Because the SPs will be putting together and practicing all exam activities for the first time during this session, consider focusing your attention during the initial round of interviews on each SP's performance with particular attention to each SP's affect and other expressions of the emotional aspects of the case. Then in the second round of encounters, all the SPs will have another opportunity to make any adjustments to their portrayals that you suggest after having observed their first practice encounter. Remember that your focus on portrayal during the initial round of practice encounters is your unspoken intention. You want the SPs to be equally focused on all of the tasks: performing, filling out and comparing checklists, writing and reviewing their comments for feedback after each encounter, and going over the observing SPs' notes.

Checklist completion. During the first round of encounters, the performing SP and the person who does the interview (in the role of the medical student) are the only ones who will be filling out the checklists and writing comments *after* the encounters. The performing SP will practice filling out her checklist on a computer. All observing SPs (and the observing SP coach, if there is an assistant) will

- fill out the printed checklists *during* the encounter, and at the same time, make notes on their observations next to the appropriate items.
- practice writing comments in the from-the-patient's-perspective section of the checklist about each interaction *after* the clinical encounter, using general and case-specific written feedback guidelines (see Appendix A6) and a list of descriptors that you and/or the SPs have created. (For more details, see Training the SPs to Give Effective Written Feedback later in this chapter on p. 215.)

Of course, comments can only be written *after* an encounter because they are a summation from the patient's perspective of the entire experience. Remember, this is the first time the SPs are practicing writing feedback to the students. Therefore, although you are timing the encounters during this session so that the SPs begin to get a feel for the exam timeframe, I suggest giving them as much time as they need to write the comments during this round. This will give them a chance to practice carefully formulating what they want to say to the student without being worried about the clock just yet.

The Second Round of Encounters

During the second round, your focus will be on all aspects of the SPs' performances, including their checklist accuracy and the quality of their written comments. Consistent accuracy on checklists should be uppermost in your mind. This will be the first time in training that the SPs will be experiencing the phenomenon of trying to remember checklist items after having filled out checklists on multiple other encounters (their own and the other SPs' practice encounters). The challenge at this time is for them not to confuse the present encounter with previous ones.

Portrayal. Consider starting the second round with your weakest performer. This will ensure that, if needed, you will have enough time to work on performance concerns and not risk running out of time for that SP at the end of the session.

Checklist completion. During the second round of encounters, everyone will perform the case, then fill out checklists and write comments after the encounter within the exam timeframe.

At this point in Training Session Three, all of the SPs should be comfortable and ready to practice everything as it will occur in the CPX. I recommend waiting until this point in this session to require the SPs to complete the checklist in the time allotted. If you put this kind of pressure on them too early in the process, it can produce unnecessary anxiety, causing them to focus on speed rather than on accuracy.

A final reminder. At the conclusion of the practice session, remind the SPs about the date of the Practice Exam and have them sign up for an equal number of specific administrations in the CPX examination schedule. Remember that the backup person you might need will come from the rotating SP who is on call for each day's exam.

This is a final commitment. Describe how you would like the SPs to handle any changes in schedule that might arise because of illness or other extenuating circumstances. Explicitly ask the SPs to call you immediately if anything occurs that would prevent them from keeping their commitment to perform in the CPX. This is why you hired an extra SP during recruitment, as backup. Let the SPs know that they will be getting a confirmation letter during Training Session Four. Each letter will include the dates of the SPs' performances as well as an estimate of the their total remuneration if there are no changes to the schedule.

Preparation of the SPs for Training Session Four

Think of Training Session Four as the first of two dress rehearsals of the SPs' performances. This dress rehearsal is a case-specific practice session in which an uninitiated clinician will verify the SPs' authenticity in playing the patient case. Only the SPs performing the same case will participate in this session. Consider the Practice Exam as the final dress rehearsal involving all the SPs for all of the cases, all the coaches, and all the administrative support staff who arrive on the same day at the same time to practice together for the first time before the actual examination with the medical students, which occurs at a later date. Even though you will do a Practice Exam, I suggest that you also rehearse all of your SPs during Training Session Four as close as possible to the actual exam protocol.

Advise the SPs to Come to Training Session Four in Full Make-Up Dressed as the Patient

You want to see how everyone has interpreted what their make-up will look like and how they will be dressed for the exam if they are not required to be in a patient gown. Do not assume that because you have discussed these details with the SPs that they will necessarily come as you have envisioned them. However, seeing them in their final ensemble gives you an opportunity to go over any changes you would like them to make in their physical appearance before the Practice Exam. For example, you might want a particular SP who is not having a physical exam but who is portraying a depressed patient to wear something similar to what they were wearing at the Session Four dress rehearsal, but in a darker or more muted color.

As far as make-up is concerned, this includes not only the regular cosmetic make-up that many women wear but also special make-up needed to simulate the patient case, for example, jaundice, pallor, bruises, any kind of moulage (e.g., scars, wounds, dressings with blood, bandages), fake IV lines, sprayed-on bourbon (for a patient who is abusing alcohol), and so on.

All the effects that compose the total impression of the patient in the case—external (what can be seen, smelled, touched on the patient) and internal (the psychological, emotional, intellectual "make-up" of the patient)—should be evident to the uninitiated clinician who will assist you, taking on the role of the medical student, in this final training session. The clinician will then be able to experience and respond to the comprehensive effect of the patient and give you and the SPs feedback on the results of your efforts.

Preview Training Session Four Activities

Let the SPs know that they will each perform one timed, video-recorded encounter with a primary care clinician who is not familiar with their case.

Inform the SPs that they will fill out checklists when they are performing as well as when they are observing, within the exam timeframe, on recall, after each encounter during Training Session Four.

When the SPs are not performing, they will be in the monitoring room observing the timed performance of their fellow SPs. For observation and recall practice, all SPs will be filling out all their checklists as if they were filling them out during an actual exam, that is, one checklist for every encounter, on recall, one after another, within the time allotted for each activity in an actual exam.

The Coach's Preparation for Session Four and the Practice Exam

Prepare a Letter of Confirmation to Give to Each SP During Training Session Four

The letter should include

- the date, time, and place of the Practice Exam.
- dates of the CPX administrations that the SP has signed up for.
- an estimate of the SP's total remuneration for training and performances.

Confirm the Appointments for Each Clinician Scheduled to Participate in Training Session Four

If, during the fourth training session, you will use business card/labels, it is a nice touch to prepare the labels for this session with the name of the health care professional who is scheduled to work with the SPs.

Continue Recruitment of Residents for the Practice Exam

TRAINING THE SPs TO GIVE EFFECTIVE WRITTEN FEEDBACK

Because giving feedback to the medical students during their Clinical Practice Examination is so beneficial—and because training the SPs to give effective feedback is so essential in Training Session Three and in the SPs' training in general—I have addressed this topic on its own here.

The Rationale for Giving the Medical Students Feedback

From the medical students' point of view, receiving feedback on their interaction skills with patients can be more difficult than getting feedback on other types of skills, such as their physical exam skills for instance. Why? Because communication skills are intimately tied up with how the students perceive themselves as people. It is the difference between being told how to hold an ophthalmoscope so that the student can get a better view of the retina versus being told how to more effectively address the patient's feelings so that the student can better show the empathy she is feeling and thus create better rapport with the patient. One is an objective skill to be learned, the other personal and subjective. By the way, being able to communicate effectively with patients is a skill most students think they already have. As one student put it, "I can't have done poorly on the PPI. I got into medical school, didn't I? I've been talking to people all my life." But, the truth is that talking to patients requires additional, special skills—skills that are not always intuitive but that can be taught and learned very effectively. For some medical students, the "Ah ha!" or sudden awareness of the truth about their communication skills comes as the SPs help them realize how the patient perceives their actions and what the patient's needs really are. This is the beginning of the students' understanding that they must focus on the patient's perspective and concerns, as much as they do on their own needs and desires to solve the patient's medical problem.

The more inexperienced the student the more eager he is to receive feedback, because novices are not expected to be able to perform proficiently. However, once the novice begins to grow in expertise—either in actuality or in his own mind—the more difficult it becomes for many to hear about areas of inadequacy in their clinical performances. Still, if the feedback is given sensitively by the SPs, the vast majority of students continue to want to know how they are coming across to the very people they are in the profession of helping to get well. This is the psychological context into which the SPs enter when sharing their observations with the students.

Of course, the manner in which the SP gives the feedback also has something to do with the way the student receives it. When the SPs give feedback well, the students frequently comment that this is the area in the encounter where they learned the most. So the SPs' giving effective feedback—on a specific set of communication skills rather than being solely influenced by their like or dislike of the student—is a real service to the students' learning and is something they cannot get as authentically anywhere else.

Getting regular, effective feedback is critical to learning and behavior change. However, students, like practicing health care professionals in general, rarely receive objective feedback from their patients. What the health care professional usually hears is either praise, if the patient was happy with the outcome of his interaction with the doctor, or complaint, if the patient did not like the way he was treated or was displeased for some other reason. Although praise may make the recipient happy and criticism upset him, this kind of nonspecific feedback is not beneficial in terms of helping the clinician to understand what in his behavior might have caused the patient to perceive him in a given way.

Imagine the difference it can make then to a student to understand the specifics of how her behavior is being perceived by the patient. The contribution the SP makes to a student's learning comes from (a) sharing his detailed perception of how the patient he is portraying has experienced working with the student and (b) eliciting from the student, or offering, suggestions for how the student might alter her approach so that she communicates more of what she intends during her exchanges with her patients.

Now to look at the other side of the coin: When we hire new SPs, they are likely to be unskilled at giving effective feedback. It takes time and practice to become good at giving feedback, so the longer your SPs are with you the better they will become at it. Eventually, you will find that most of the SPs—even those you think may never be really good at giving feedback—after working with the students and being coached again and again, finally do learn, and one day will surprise you at how skillful they have become.

The Role of the SPs in Giving the Medical Students Feedback

In order to fully develop this critical skill, the SPs need to understand the value of giving feedback to the student. First let's look at how feedback works in general, then how it applies to the SP who will be giving feedback to the medical student from the patient's point of view.

Only the Persons Interacting With Each Other Can Legitimately Say What Is Transpiring Between the Two of Them

The assumption that how an interaction appeared to an observer is how the participants actually experienced it is a common fallacy. To truly understand what transpired in an interaction, the observer must check out her assumptions with the participants in order to be certain about what took place on an emotional level individually for each of them—and in the interaction between them.

This principle applies equally in the medical setting. No *observer* of an encounter between patient and doctor can give feedback about what happened between them that is as valid as that of the persons who were engaged in the encounter itself—even if the observer was in the room where the interaction took place. SPs are unique in this regard in that they can be trained to give objective feedback (about the patient they portrayed) from their own perspective as the person who played the part of that patient. Real patients always have feelings about their interactions with their doctors, but they rarely know how to express those feelings in ways that would be helpful to the clinician.

Worse yet is the assumption that how one perceives a student's performance on a video recording or via a monitor is how the patient experienced the student. Video recordings, because they are two dimensional, are a step removed from the reality of the interaction and are valid only as a record of *what* the student said and did, not of *how* the student came across to the patient.

As coaches we too need to be careful not to overstep this boundary. Once our SPs can satisfactorily give feedback to us in our interactions with them in training, we must trust their judgment about their interactions with the students, even if our perception differs from theirs. So long as the SPs can articulate why they are assessing the student's interpersonal skills in a particular way—based on the guidelines we have trained them to use—it is the SPs' judgments on which we must rely.

Standardized Patients Can Be More Objective Than Real Patients

Unlike certain real patients, SPs have no ax to grind with the medical profession, no real illness to deal with, and, therefore, no motives of self-interest when giving the student feedback, as well as no need to make themselves feel better by merely discharging emotional reactions.

Standardized Patients Can Be Trained to Give Feedback That Supports Learning and Behavior Change

Getting feedback on their interaction skills from the SPs may be the only time during their training that the medical students receive constructive feedback from the point of view of the patient. However, to give feedback that is beneficial to these students, the SPs must be trained in how to shape their remarks so that they will be heard by the student—heard and integrated, rather than rejected and perhaps ignored.

If the SP is expected to give feedback, but is not specifically trained to do so, the result can do more harm than good. The following are examples of undesirable situations that can occur when untrained SPs are asked to give feedback. Untrained SPs might make comments that

- contradict what the faculty are trying to teach the students.
- cause the student doctor to become defensive when he reads inept, unhelpful comments such as
  "I wouldn't come back to this student because he doesn't know his medicine."
  "I didn't like this student. He's too unprofessional."
- are about something the student doctor cannot change, such as
  "I think this student is too young to be taking care of an old lady like me."

When an untrained SP gives such feedback, his effort is in vain—or even harmful—and the students are likely to discount whatever else the SP has to say, even if it is valid. (Before sending out the SPs' written comments to the students, always review them to make sure the content is appropriate and clear in its intent.)

SPs Can Help Students Improve Their Communication Skills

Whether or not there is a formal doctor–patient communication program in your medical school curriculum, anytime that SPs are used for teaching or assessment purposes, they can provide an opportunity for the students to learn—from the patient's point of view—about the effectiveness of their interaction. The SPs can help medical students understand that the way they interact with the patient not only affects how the patient perceives the student but also how forthcoming, confident, and willing the patient might be

- to share everything that is pertinent to his condition, particularly sensitive information that the patient might feel uncomfortable talking about with someone he does not trust (for example, the use of drugs in an adolescent, fear of cardiovascular problems if a patient's brother has just died of a heart attack, and so on).

- to follow lifestyle changes suggested by the student.

- to adhere to medical recommendations made by the student (such as, follow-through on tests, filling of prescriptions, taking of medications).

On high-stakes examinations such as the CPX, patient–physician interaction skills are typically built into the checklist itself, requiring the SPs to rate the student on a number of communication items using dichotomous (yes/no) choices or a Likert (range of responses) scale. But a numerical score on a cluster of interaction items does not help the student understand her own communication skills in the same way that specific SP comments can.

In fact, the SPs' written comments sometimes capture aspects of a student's behavior that are not found in the specific PPI items. Because this kind of information can be very helpful to faculty who will be doing remediation, and because students maintain that one of the most powerful aspects of working with standardized patients is the feedback they get from them, it is well worth considering the incorporation of written SP comments into every summative evaluation—as well as into any other situation where verbal feedback from the SP is not feasible or appropriate.

Practical Suggestions for Training SPs to Give Written Feedback

In the following section, you will find principles and practical suggestions for training your SPs to give effective written feedback to the medical students.

Select a Few Principles for Giving Feedback

Always Have the SPs Offer Feedback From the Perspective of the Patient

Give the SPs guidelines on how to let the students know what it was like to be the patient they were portraying. The uniqueness and strength of the feedback given by the SPs come from their having experienced being the patient. The SP often has a better, more universal understanding of the patient than did the real patient on whom the case is based. The SP can be more objective about the patient's experiences because she is not facing all of the actual issues the real patient was dealing with. Because the SP will have been trained to look for, and reflect back to the students, specific interpersonal and communication skills that affected the patient in identifiable ways, the SP's feedback can provide the student with insight about her own interpersonal style.

No one else can give as accurate a description of the patient's experience as the SP—not the other students, not the faculty facilitator, nor the student in the interaction with the patient, because no one but the SP was in the skin of the patient. No doubt everyone will have an opinion about what was going on with the patient, but only the SP can say for certain.

Encourage the SPs to Share Their Insight Using the Patient's Pseudonym When Giving Feedback

For example, "*Derrick* felt such-and-such . . ." not "*I* felt such-and-such. . . ."

By talking about what the patient experienced, the SP allies himself with the student, sharing with her as a colleague an event that both of them experienced together—an event in which the SP played the part of the patient and the student played the part of the doctor.

Make Sure That the SPs Do Not Give Feedback on the Medical Issues of the Case

The SP should not give feedback that is more appropriate for faculty to give, such as correcting the student's diagnosis of the patient's medical condition, giving medical information, or telling the students questions they should have asked or physical examination maneuvers they should have done. Only the faculty have the authority to give this kind of information to the medical students. Remind the SPs that their area of expertise is in how the patient experienced the clinical encounter with the student. Be sure that the SPs explicitly understand that discussing medical issues is an easy trap to innocently fall into because, as a result of their training, the standardized patients sometimes *do* understand more medical information about the patient they are portraying than the medical students do.

Make Sure the SPs Have <u>at Least One Key Response</u> to Use in Giving Feedback

A *key response* is a bit of information related to the evaluation objectives that are critical to the case and that will work in feedback no matter what happened in the encounter. Key responses are an important aid for the SPs who cannot take notes while performing the case and sometimes draw a blank when feeling pressured to come up with something to write immediately after the encounter regarding the student's interaction with them. Therefore, having several key responses available for the SPs to use in order to break the ice gives them the safety to confidently put in writing what they have just experienced in the clinical encounter. Make these key responses available throughout their training so that the SPs get acquainted with them for whenever they cannot come up with anything else to write about. (For sample key responses on the Gomez case, see Appendix A6, Guidelines for Giving Written Feedback.)

Use the "Club Sandwich" Technique in the Feedback

At the beginning, middle, and end of their feedback, encourage the SPs to write positive comments to shore up the student's confidence. These genuinely positive affirmations of the students' efforts help them build confidence in their ability to master the skills they are practicing and prepare them to more readily accept what the SPs have to say about the parts of their interaction skills that need adjustment. The SPs can start out sharing positive observations about the overall encounter, including the *positive intentions* that the SP sensed the student was trying to express, even if his attempts were not successful. Or the SP might start with a generic comment about the case, letting the student know that "this was a difficult case that anyone, except the most seasoned physician, would find hard to deal with."

Between these positive comments, have the SPs sandwich no more than two or three constructive suggestions based on the learning objectives built into the case. (These are the key responses just referred to.)

The notion of writing feedback that encompasses what the student is doing well, along with what he can improve, is intended to reinforce the principle that feedback is not just about recognizing and correcting unskillful student behavior; it is also about reinforcing the proficiencies of the students so that they become aware of the *effective* means they might already be using intuitively. The more conscious the students become about the effects of their behavior on their patients during their interactions, the more likely they will (a) continue to use the skills that are working for them and (b) strive to improve behaviors that were having adverse effects on their patients—of which they had been unaware.

Discuss Specific Behaviors—Not Attitudes, Personalities, or Assumed Motivations

Encourage the SPs to back up any general comments they make with details. In other words, they are *not* to write in generalities, such as this actual comment from an SP: "Jerry liked your bedside manner and thought you were very professional." Nor are they to comment on abstract ideas or assumptions about student behavior or on anything the student cannot change. For instance, the following is *not* a helpful suggestion: "Jerry would have opened up more about his sexual practices if you hadn't been so judgmental (or so pushy, so annoying, so young, so . . .)."

Instead, encourage the SPs to share what the medical student specifically said or did that caused the patient to perceive the student as judgmental. The student needs to know what being judgmental means. Here is a more helpful way to let the student know what caused the patient to clam up: "Jerry would have opened up more about his sexual practices if you had asked him how he found himself having to survive on the street, rather than referring to him as a prostitute."

Let the Students Know What They Could Have Done Differently

The students not only need to know what they did that caused the SP to react the way he did, but they also need to know what they could have done instead to help the patient feel more comfortable in sharing his concerns. Therefore, encourage the SPs to make specific suggestions such as:

> Jerry might have felt more willing to discuss his sexual practices if you had helped him understand why you needed to know.
>
> or
>
> Jerry would have felt you cared more about him if he hadn't been interrupted every time he tried to tell his story.

Provide Other Resources for SPs to Use When Writing Comments

While keeping in mind these principles for giving feedback, here are several aids you can use to help the SPs learn how to write effective comments.

The Level of the SP's Overall Satisfaction With the Encounter

The overall satisfaction of the patient with the encounter should be item #1 on the checklist because it is the item you want the SPs to fill out before completing the rest of the checklist. In our sample case, Item #1 reads, "As Maria Gomez, rate your overall level of satisfaction with this student encounter." The explanation of this item in the guide to the checklist states,

> Your response to this item should be as "Maria Gomez"—NOT as you, the SP portraying the patient who knows what the medical student is being tested on in the checklist. The idea behind this item is to determine your overall satisfaction with the encounter immediately after the student leaves the room. It encompasses whether
>
> • you feel you would come back to this student physician for the rest of your care.

- you feel this student was or will be able to help you (in your total care). (See the first page of Appendix A5.)

This overall satisfaction item comes first on every checklist so that it can capture the SP's overall sense of the encounter right after the student leaves the room and before their feeling about the interaction is influenced by knowing how the student did on the rest of the checklist. In addition, this item effectively captures unique aspects of student behavior not found in the more specific, individual PPI items. Thus, this item can be quite useful to the SPs in their written comments. At the very least, a statement at the end of the SP's comments, stimulated by this item, can serve as a summary of the specifics the SP has brought up about his experience with the student. For example, the last comment might read, "For these reasons, I do not feel this student doctor can help me" or "For these reasons, I would definitely come back to this student doctor for the rest of my care."

Patient–Physician Interaction Checklist Items

Another resource for helping SPs with written comments are the Patient–Physician Interaction items themselves and the explanations in the guide to the checklist, which give insight into the intent and meaning behind each PPI item. Basing the written feedback on the PPI scale used in the checklist makes the job of writing comments simpler and clearer for the SPs, especially if you provide (in the guide to the checklist) parameters within which to understand and work with the items (see Appendix A5). While the SPs are filling out this section of the checklist, they can jot down notes on what comes to mind as they score each item. These notes can then trigger the comments they write.

Case Summary or "From the Patient's Perspective"

If a summary that incorporates the essence of the case from the patient's point of view is printed at the top of the comment section of the patient's checklist, the SPs can refer to it while writing their comments (see the last page of Appendix A4).

Here is another example of a from-the-patient's-perspective summary for a different checklist:

> David Matthews is concerned about missing work due to his back pain and the possibility that his back problems will have long-term effects on his physical ability. He wants the doctor to acknowledge his concern about loss of work and address his fear about this becoming a chronic condition.

Notice that the Gomez and Matthews' case summaries focus on two key issues:

- the patient's agenda.
- the patient's expectation(s) for the visit.

Create a Document That Includes Both General and Specific Guidelines for Writing Feedback

The purpose of such a document is to highlight for the SPs what you want them to remember when they are writing comments. It can include any of the suggestions already listed in this section or others that you are already coaching your SPs to use. You might want to use the Guidelines for Giving Written Feedback (see Appendix A6) in the Maria Gomez case to create something similar for your own cases as you see fit. It contains both general and case specific guidelines intended for the SPs' use during training and actual exam performances.

Create a List of Descriptors the SPs Can Use When Writing Comments

If you remember, the SPs use a list of verbs to select an action they will use in order to get what they want from the doctor when they are performing during the encounter. So too, the SPs can use a list of adjectives or descriptors as an aid for writing their individualized comments about their clinical experience with the medical student. This list of adjectives can be a valuable tool to assist the SPs when they are trying to find the right word to express the feelings they, as the patient, were experiencing during their interaction with the medical student. The list of descriptors will help them more quickly write these feedback comments in the brief time allotted after the encounter.

You can create such a list on your own, or you can do it together with your SPs. The list usually consists of two sets of adjectives—one to use when the patient's feeling was positive, the other when the feeling was uncomfortable or downright negative about something the student doctor said or did.

Using the case in this book as an example, the SP would start her written comments by completing the phrase, "As Maria Gomez, I felt..." (see the last page of Appendix A4). For any feelings she wants to share that were positive, the SP would select descriptors such as "cared for," "understood," "heard," "confident," "relieved," "satisfied," and so on. If the SP is feeling uncomfortable about anything that happened during the encounter, she could choose words such as "disregarded," "unimportant," "uncertain," "irritated," or "talked down to." Then following each of these statements, the SP should indicate the specific student behavior(s) that caused her to feel the way she just described.

One final word. Make sure that the general and case specific guidelines for giving written feedback (that you have designed for the specific case you are training) are included in the SPs' manuals so they can use them starting with this training session. They should also have these feedback guidelines, as well as a copy of the list of descriptors, in the exam room every time they perform their cases from now on, including during the Practice Exam and the actual CPX exam administrations. By having these documents at their sides, they can use them as quick references whenever the need arises.

CHAPTER TEN

Training Session Four: First Dress Rehearsal (Clinician Verification of SPs' Authenticity)

Dress rehearsals are indispensable when preparing for any complex, carefully choreographed event, like a clinical practice examination. In this context, what dress rehearsal means is an uninterrupted practice session for the SPs in the exam setting, each dressed and made up as the case requires, performing encounters in the rooms they will use during the exam. All the equipment, supplies, gowns, and sheets should be stored exactly where the SPs will find them during the exam administrations. The presenting situation and other information for the students should be in place as well. To prepare for an actual exam, you and your SPs will be doing the dress rehearsal in two phases:

- Training Session Four—final preparation, done in the context of a single case with an uninitiated clinician (in the role of the medical student) running a single encounter with each of the SPs one after another in order to verify the authenticity of their performances.
- The Practice Exam—a mock-up of an actual CPX administration in which every case and all personnel—all administrative staff, the coaches, assistant coaches, along with all the SPs from all of the cases who will be involved in the CPX—are present to practice the exam logistics. Residents (or other qualified health care trainees) serve as the examinees in place of the medical students to give the SPs and their coaches one final chance to make performance adjustments before they begin working with the students whose clinical skills the SPs will observe and document during the CPX.

227

During Training Session Four, you, your assistant, and all the SPs from a single case will observe each SP consecutively perform that individual case with a clinician who has not otherwise been involved in the training and who assumes the role of the medical student in the clinical encounter. All the encounters will take place in the exam room in which the SPs will perform during the CPX. All observations by the coach and the nonperforming SPs will take place in the monitoring room using the video monitoring equipment for the station assigned to that case. As final training proceeds, this observation protocol allows the coach an opportunity to make certain that all cameras, monitors, computers, recording equipment, and headsets are in working order under the same conditions they will be used during the actual exam.

All the cameras and furniture in each exam room should have been positioned for optimal video viewing of the examinee's (medical student's) activities throughout the entire encounter. Although all the exam rooms have been set up as they would be for an actual exam administration, during final training it sometimes becomes clear that supplies are missing, a piece of equipment is not functioning properly, or a camera needs adjustment. All of these issues can be identified and taken care of during Session Four rather than at the last minute during the Practice Exam.

Even though it is possible for you, the coach, to run this session by yourself, it is better to have someone assist you with the rotation of the SPs between the monitoring room (where the observing SPs will be situated) and the exam room (where the actual encounter will take place with the clinician).

Your assistant can make sure that the observing SPs in the monitoring room have blank checklists to work with, that they are concentrating on the performance (and not interacting with each other), and that the SP who is next in line to perform is ready to make the switch with the SP in the exam room. Having an assistant who can handle all these logistical activities frees you, as the coach, to focus on the visiting clinician, in order to

- orient her to what she will be doing during the session.
- exchange information with her on the case and the assessment goals.
- elicit her clinical impressions following each encounter.

It is also beneficial for the person who will be in charge of exam logistics to participate in at least one of the Session Four case rehearsals. This gives the exam administrator a chance to practice timing each of the encounters, along with giving cues over the intercom as they will be given to the examinees and the SPs during the CPX. Here are some examples of typical announcements:

- signaling the start of the exam over the intercom, letting the examinees know how many minutes are left in the encounter, prompting the end of the interaction with "Student doctor you are needed in the hallway."
- timing the filling out of the checklists with cues to help the SPs gauge how long they have left to complete this activity, write their comments, and re-prep their rooms (putting their guide to the checklist and feedback guidelines away, repositioning any equipment that has been moved, refolding the sheet used for draping) before the next examinee knocks on the door.

The Goal of Training Session Four

By the end of this session, all standardized patients of a given case should be ready to perform, that is, they should look, feel, and act just like a real patient. They should be 100% accurate in their performances and be able to complete all the checklists within the exam timeframe, with the goal of 100% accuracy, but with no less than an 85% overall accuracy rate.

The Training Setting

Ideally, the practice encounters with the uninitiated clinician should take place in the very exam room where the SPs will perform during the actual CPX. You and all the observing SPs will watch the encounters from the video monitoring room. You will discuss and compare the checklists with the SPs in a small conference room after the clinician has finished all of the encounters and been released.

Summary of the Training Activities

Because Training Session Four is a dress rehearsal, the timed encounters (between the clinician and each of the SPs) and filling out the checklists by all the SPs after each encounter should take place one after another with only enough time between encounters for the coach to do a short debrief with the clinician while the next SP is rotating into the exam room. After a complete interaction with each of the SPs, the clinician is free to depart while the coach and the SPs spend the rest of the session reviewing the checklists from each encounter.

Reminders

There Should Be at Least 1 Day Between Session Three and Session Four

Sometimes it is not possible to follow the guideline of scheduling each training session approximately 1 week apart. For various reasons you might need to schedule two sessions in the same week. If that becomes necessary, give the SPs at least 24 hours between training sessions—in other words, enough time to integrate what they have learned from the previous session.

A Clinician Who Is Not Familiar With the Case Should Have Been Recruited for This Session

The clinician you have recruited should come to this fourth and final training session knowing no more about the case itself than the medical students will during the CPX. (For the kind of information to share with the clinician about what he or she will be doing during this session, see on the following page: Topics to discuss with the clinician—and when.) The clinician should be suited to the case and to the type of assessment you are doing. For example, if you were testing medical students on general clinical practice skills, a primary care physician would be a good choice of clinician. However, if you were working in a nursing school on a clinical exam to certify pediatric nurse practitioners, the clinician would ideally be a nurse practitioner with a background in that specialty. (For more details, see Start Recruiting Clinicians for Training Session Four, under Coach's Preparation in chapter 7.)

The following considerations are important when working with the clinician in Session Four:

A Formula for Determining How Long the Clinician Needs to Be Present During Session Four Training

Multiply the length of the station plus the length of time allotted for filling out the checklist plus a few minutes to discuss the encounter with the clinician times the number of SPs to be interviewed. For example, suppose you have an exam with 15-minute stations and postencounter write-ups of 10 minutes. You want to spend 5 minutes talking with the clinician after each encounter with each of three SPs. Here is how to calculate the amount of time the clinician needs to spend with you during this final training session:

$$15 + 10 + 5 = 30 \text{ minutes} \times 3 \text{ SPs} = 90 \text{ minutes} (1\frac{1}{2} \text{ hours})$$

Topics to Discuss With the Clinician—and When

Prior to this session, when you are recruiting the clinician, discuss only basic facts about the case.   The basic facts include the age and presenting symptoms of the patient, such as a 42-year-old man with recurring back pain. You will also want to give details on who the clinician will be working with, and that she will be

- following the same protocol as the medical students (to help determine if the case instructions and all other directions are clear).
- sharing with you her impressions about how each standardized patient came across to her. You might consider asking the clinician questions such as these: Did the SP appear to be symptomatically convincing and factually accurate? Were the SP's simulated physical findings and his corresponding reactions and affect realistic? Did the interaction with the SP feel as genuine as interactions with real patients? If not, why not? (These impressions that the clinician has of the SP are key to helping you work with the SPs on any adjustments that their performances might need.)
- serially interviewing each of the SPs-in-training.

During this session, before the clinician encounters the first SP, go over all activities in which the clinician will participate.   You will also want to show her the student instructions and presenting situation for the station.

Do not give other details about the case until after the first encounter. Let the clinician know why you would prefer not to share any other information about the case with her until she has worked with the first SP. Ask her to give you feedback on her untutored impressions of the SP experience, including whether or not the instructions to the medical student were clear and provided enough of the right information to adequately deal with the patient challenge.

Record all of the Encounters and Save all of the SPs' Checklists

As in all the training sessions, the video recordings and checklists can be used to review the SPs' performance progress and by the CPX advisory committee as needed.

Session Four Training Activities (Estimated Time: 3 hours)

The Clinician's Activities

Once you have shared an overview of the session's activities and given the clinician the student instructions to read, do the following:

Have the Clinician Conduct a Timed Run-Through of the Case With Each SP

The timing during this rehearsal is the same timing you will use during the actual exam administrations for both the encounter and the write-up the students will be doing while the SPs are filling out checklists. Practicing the timing of each SP's performance during this session helps give them a sense of what it will be like to perform one encounter after another and to fill out checklist after checklist during the actual exam. It also indicates whether what is being asked of the students is realistic in the given timeframe. If you find that the experienced clinician has trouble accomplishing what is expected, the students will certainly have difficulty. It is still not too late to have the CPX advisory committee consider adjusting the requirements according to this new information.

Encourage the Clinician to Be as Thorough as Possible Within the Timeframe Without Trying to Do a Perfect Performance

Ask the experienced clinician instead to try to "think like an examinee"— in other words, to work with the SPs at the examinees' level of training, for example, beginning fourth-year medical students who are expected to do everything by the book. You can also let the clinician know that you would prefer she not do everything flawlessly. These directives set the tone of the session in two important ways:

- Most clinicians are a little anxious about being video monitored, let alone having their performance recorded. Making the clinician aware that you prefer that she *not* do a perfect performance lets her off the hook, so to speak, so that she does not feel that her recorded performances have to be exemplary.
- Your instructions let the clinician know that the focus of her interactions with the SPs is supposed to be on the SPs and that the session is about giving *them* practice. In other words, the clinician can be most helpful in putting the SPs through their paces by *not* doing everything she might normally do. This kind of imperfect encounter challenges the SPs to remember what was done or *not* done when they fill out the checklist.

After Each Encounter, Discuss the Clinician's Observations of Each SP's Performance

In another nearby room, while all the SPs are filling out the checklist on the encounter, you will have time to go over any observations the clinician has made regarding the SP's presentation and portrayal of the case.

Assist the Clinician in Varying Her Approach With Each SP

Because the clinician will know details about the case after working with the first SP, it is important to help her give the *other* SPs as thorough and as fresh a clinical experience as possible. You do not want the clinician simply repeating what she did in her first encounter with each of the other SPs. Showing the clinician the checklist can be quite helpful. You can suggest examples of good and poor physical exam techniques to use during successive interviews, questions to leave out, or give her permission to follow a line of questioning regarding anything the patient might bring up that the clinician would not ordinarily pursue. Such suggestions can aid the clinician in thinking of ways to creatively and realistically keep the successive SP encounters new and challenging.

Another suggestion that often helps clinicians vary their performances from SP to SP is to ask them to think of a particular medical student or resident they have supervised and to try to duplicate some of their behaviors. Encourage the clinicians to make some of the errors their medical students or residents make: stumble, ask questions in a disorganized fashion, think out loud, or use the clipboard for notetaking as a crutch. In other words, encourage the clinicians to use behaviors they have observed that hinder the establishment of rapport with the patient.

Here are two examples of what I mean. In regard to the adolescent case referred to earlier, another issue that Brittany Eisler has with her parents is that they are not happy with the grades she is getting in school. After the first dress rehearsal interview, in which the adolescent medicine physician showed real empathy with *Brittany's* perception of the situation, I asked the physician, in the next interview, to try to get Brittany to see things from her *parents'* point of view (an approach we had seen a number of students take with the patient in previous exams).

In a different practice encounter, rather than skillfully leading into the sensitive questions about drugs, alcohol, and sex, I suggested that the clinician simply blurt out questions to Brittany with or without effective transitions. Instead of normalizing the situation as she had in the first encounter ("You are at the age when young people sometimes experiment with drugs and alcohol. Are any of your friends doing that? [pause]. What about you—have you tried any of these things?"), I requested that the clinician lead into these questions with something less skillful, without any transition as if the medical student had just gotten to that part of the list-of-things-to-cover-with-an-adolescent: "So, you're getting a C average in school. Okay. . . .So are you sexually active?" By asking these sensitive questions, using no transition, and altering her approach to one or another of the challenges built into the case, the clinician was able to provide different performance experiences for each of the SPs during the dress rehearsal. These contrasting approaches required the SPs to handle answering the questions on drugs, alcohol, and sex in different ways, depending on the rapport and trust Brittany felt with the physician.

While the SPs Are Filling Out Their Checklists, Give the Students' Interstation Exercise (Postencounter Write-Up) to the Clinician to Complete After the First Encounter

By completing this exercise, the clinician will not only bring to your attention any items or activities that might need clarification or additional information but will also provide you with supporting information for the key to the interstation exercise, which can be used to grade it (see Appendix A8, Interstation Exercise, and Appendix A9, Interstation Exercise Key.)

Another way to approach this activity is to ask the clinician, before showing her the interstation exercise, "Now that you've experienced working with the patient, what do *you* think would be an appropriate or reasonable written follow-up for a student to do after seeing this patient?"

To cite the Brittany Eisler case again—the physician who did final training on this case thought the interstation exercise we were using was "trivial." She felt it would be more beneficial to have the students do the assessment and plan (the "A" and "P" of a SOAP note—a typical format physicians use to make chart notes on a patient) and/or ask such questions as "What additional information do you need to get from Brittany's parents in order to decide on your next steps?" or "Because issues of confidentiality are raised here, how much information, if any, does the student need to share with Brittany's parents? Why?/Why not?" or "What are the options for helping Brittany get reproductive health care without her parents' knowledge?" and so on.

These are the kinds of issues that emerge during the fourth training session and warrant the attention of the CPX advisory committee—even at the 11th hour. The physician's feedback on the Brittany Eisler interstation exercise was eye opening and gave the committee another perspective to consider.

Show the Checklist to the Clinician After the Second Encounter

Elicit any suggestions the clinician might have for its improvement. Find out if she feels there is something critical that should be added to the checklist or if there are items on the checklist that she thinks are superfluous. Always explore the reasoning behind any suggestions.

Discuss the Realism of Each SP's Performance and Answer Any Questions That Might Have Arisen for the Clinician About the Case

Do this after *every* encounter so that you can give feedback to each SP later. Do *not* share this information with the SP at this time (unless you determine that the clinician's participation in giving the feedback is necessary, such as adjusting a simulated physical finding). Otherwise, protect the clinician's time and wait to go over these details after she has gone.

If, however, the clinician is friendly to the process, understands the goals of the case, is eager to share her ideas with the SPs, and has the time—then, after all the SPs have been through their practice encounters, bring them together for the clinician to give them her feedback.

Do Not Change the Facts or Emphasis of the Case

In contrast to the clinicians who have written an SP case, or reviewed a written version, clinicians who experience the case firsthand through working with a trained SP, often discover—and are quite passionate about—changes they believe would improve the case. Understandably so. They are the ones who have actually experienced how the case plays out, so they can be quite convincing in their rationale for making necessary changes. However, this is not the moment to incorporate new ideas into the case. At this point, certain kinds of changes can be disconcerting to the SPs, or even potentially damaging to the overall evaluation structure of the clinical examination.

Take Notes on Any Suggestions the Clinician Gives

If the clinician has ideas about the case that are much different from those you have been working with, the most prudent action is to simply take notes on the clinician's ideas and let her know that you will take all suggestions to the CPX advisory committee for their consideration. A clinician who has come to the case without prior knowledge *and* who now has actual experience with how the SP case unfolds often has insights that are important and sometimes require only minor changes that can be easily made prior to the start of an exam. Here is an example of one such situation:

> In the case of a middle-age man with abdominal pain, the guide to the checklist instructed the SPs to give credit on the item that read, "The student checked for rebound tenderness," only if the student *both* performed the maneuver *and* asked the SP if he felt more pain when the student was pushing in or when he suddenly let go.
>
> During final training, when the SP did not give the clinician credit for this item because she did not *ask* him when he felt more pain, the

clinician responded that she always *watches* the patient's facial expression as verification for when the patient experiences the greatest pain. This completely valid, nonverbal form of checking rebound tenderness became a concern of the CPX advisory committee—and the guidelines were changed just prior to the start of the exam.

*After the Final Encounter, Thank the Clinician and Release Her
From the Session*

The rest of the session will not require the expertise of the clinician. It will consist of follow-up activities between you and the standardized patients, based on the clinician's encounters with the SPs. You will also be preparing the SPs for the Practice Exam and for their first performances in the CPX itself.

The Assistant's and Observing SPs' Activities

Your assistant will manage the rotation of each SP, out of the monitoring room into the exam room, to perform the case without making the change obvious to the clinician. In addition, the assistant will take care of the following details:

- *Letting the SPs know the rotation schedule and the procedures for changing places prior to the clinician's arrival.* The first encounter for the clinician is usually the most thorough and the one that is the freshest because the clinician is newly uncovering the issues of the case. Keep this in mind when determining the rotation schedule and deciding which SP should start the session. For this initial interaction, you might want to select the person with the least experience as an SP, to make sure that she gets the clinician's first encounter with the case. Or you can select the SP who gives the most exemplary performance, the one that you want to set the tone for the other SPs.

- *Making sure that all SPs are in make-up, dressed appropriately (if the case does not have a physical exam) or in a patient gown.*

- *Ensuring that the first SP is in the exam room ready to perform as soon as the clinician has been briefed by the coach.*

- *Making certain that the SPs who are not performing are in place in the monitoring room.* In order for the encounter to be a true simulation of the exam situation, no one but the clinician and the SP playing the patient should be in the exam room during the encounters in this session. However, all the observing SPs should watch each encounter from the monitoring room.

- *Seeing to it that all SPs, whether performing or observing, fill out a checklist in the exam timeframe immediately following each encounter.*

The Coach's Activities

If you have an assistant, your primary responsibilities during this training session are to work with the clinician (in the manner just described), to make any adjustments in the SPs' performances that you feel are warranted, and to lead the checklist discussion with the SPs after the clinician has finished doing one encounter with each of them. Here are some specific recommendations regarding these responsibilities:

Go Over Any Performance or Case Issues That You or the Clinician Observed During This Rehearsal

Because you have previously been so involved in the training, interviewing, coaching, and organizing, this opportunity to sit in the monitoring room and watch an uninitiated clinician interact with the patients one after another can provide new insight into the case, how it is playing, and how everything is working together. These insights can be on SP performance issues, checklist design, or case inconsistencies or oversights.

Fill Out a Checklist <u>During</u> Each Encounter

Take notes on anything that happens during the encounter that leads you to give the clinician credit for an item. Also write down whether each physical examination maneuver on the checklist was done correctly or incorrectly. Finally, record anything that the SP does in performance that you want to discuss, such as the patient's affect that might need coaching, any adjustments regarding level of pain, which items were volunteered, together with *what led up* to giving away the information.

As you have already found, your notes are an important aid in helping the SPs recall and verify questions, answers, and actions that took place during the encounter that led them to the decisions they made in filling out the checklist.

Do <u>Not</u> Compare Checklists After Each Encounter

Comparing checklists right after filling them out would be ideal, but this means that the SPs would not have the advantage of experiencing one complete encounter after another. Also, the clinician would have to wait too long between encounters while everyone completes an activity in which she is not involved. Therefore, postpone going over the checklists until after all the encounters have been completed.

Unless you feel a need to go over the simulation of a physical finding based on your observation of the case or on the recommendation of the clinician, as soon as all the SPs have performed one complete encounter (and while you say goodbye to the clinician), they can change back into street clothes before reviewing the checklists.

Review Each Set of Checklists, Encounter by Encounter, in Reverse Order, Starting With the Most Recent

Using this rule of thumb, the first checklist to review will be from the last encounter—the freshest and most immediate experience. The checklist from the last encounter is the one that will potentially have SP errors, which may be due to confusing one encounter with another. Working backwards from the most recent encounter has another advantage in that the final checklist you review will be from the first encounter of the session. Even though the first encounter is the most difficult one about which to recall details during this review, it is usually the one for which the SPs are most accurate in filling out the checklist, simply because it was the first one that everyone completed.

Use Your Notes on the Checklists to Resolve All Discrepancies

The importance of the notes you made on your checklists during the encounters will be particularly apparent as you review the SPs' checklists from encounters that are one or two steps removed from the immediacy of the experience. Just as you have been doing, focus primarily on items where there is disagreement or where you feel an emphasis is necessary, based on the SPs' previous performances.

Preparation of the SPs for the Practice Exam

Putting on a full practice exam helps assure that all of the elements are integrated and running smoothly before the first actual exam administration. Additionally, during this mock exam, the SPs get a realistic feel for the CPX and what it will be like to see one examinee after another.

There should be at least 1 or 2 days between Training Session Four and the Practice Exam so that the SPs can integrate what they have learned and you have enough time to make final preparations. The Practice Exam should be scheduled no earlier than a week, but no fewer than 2 days, before the beginning of the CPX so that what everyone has learned from the Practice Exam is still fresh, and there are still a couple of days to take care of any logistical problems that were uncovered during the Practice Exam session. In preparation for the Practice Exam:

Distribute Individualized Confirmation Letters to the SPs at the End of This Training Session

This letter should specify the date of the Practice Exam, the SPs' performance schedule, and the total compensation they will receive for their participation in all CPX activities. The total payment for the SPs reflects what each will receive for training, the Practice Exam, and their number of performances in the CPX, based on the sign-up schedule completed by the SPs at the end of Training Session Three.

Remind the SPs to Let You Know as Soon as Possible if They Cannot Perform as Scheduled

This allows you or your assistant time to contact the backup SP to cover for them in their absence.

Go Over the Practice Exam Protocols With the SPs

Let the SPs know how the Practice Exam procedures differ from the CPX. The primary difference is that instead of only one SP being present for each case, *all of the SPs will be present for all of the cases*. (See chapter 12 for more details on the Practice Exam.) This mock exam gives everyone an opportunity to put it all together logistically and make final adjustments before the first group of students arrives for the CPX.

Go Over Your Own CPX Guidelines for Standardized Patients

Whether this is a formal document or an informal discussion, it is wise (if you have time) to review the CPX guidelines for the SPs in the relative calm of this fourth and final training session so that they are familiar with all that will be expected of them and can ask questions before the Practice Exam. These guidelines can include such information as arrival time, schedule, logistics, parking, and so on. You might also want to review the specific procedures to be followed by the SPs during both the Practice Exam and the CPX, such as:

Getting in Touch With the Coach or Proctor During the Examination

Depending on the technology you have available, while the students are outside the exam room completing their postencounter write ups, the SPs can either use the private paging system from their individual rooms or simply wave at the camera to indicate a need, such as help with a checklist that is not showing up on the computer or the return of a reflex hammer or penlight that the previous medical student took out of the exam room.

Paying Attention to the Intercom Announcements

Some of the announcements are specifically meant for the SPs, such as the 1-minute warning they will get before the start of the next encounter so that the SPs will have time to submit their checklist, straighten out equipment, fold the drape sheet, and get into place.

Staying in Their Rooms at the Break and at the End of the Exam

SPs must remain in their rooms until they hear the announcement letting them know that all of the examinees have cleared the hallways.

Discuss the Intermittent Monitoring and Feedback Procedures With the SPs

You should intermittently monitor and give regular feedback to all the SPs throughout the Practice Exam and throughout all of the administrations of the CPX. It is important that the SPs know that this monitoring has nothing to do with your impression of how they did during training. The SPs need to understand—and trust—that if you had any reservations about their ability to consistently perform up to CPX standards, you would have already let them know.

The reason for the intermittent monitoring of SP performances throughout the exam is to help the SPs maintain the high standards they have achieved during training. The natural tendency when performing the same case for an extended period of time is for the SPs' performances to drift and their concentration to waiver. Research has shown that the SPs maintain higher accuracy throughout the whole of the examination if their coaches do two things: (a) randomly monitor each SP's performances during every exam administration, taking notes on performance errors and filling out checklists during the encounters and (b) give the SPs feedback on their observations and compare their checklists with those that the SPs have completed. This should be done at regular intervals, such as at the breaks and at the end of each exam administration (Wallace, 1999). If this monitoring and giving feedback is done consistently and the recruitment and training protocols found in this book are followed, the accuracy of your standardized patients' performances and checklists will likely be higher than the SP accuracies reported in the literature to date. (For a complete list of research related to this topic, see Heine, 2003.)

The Coach's Preparation for the Practice Exam

Confirm the participation of the SPs, trainers, and administrative staff on the scheduled date of the Practice Exam. If necessary, continue recruitment of residents (or other appropriate health care trainees) to play the part of examinees during the Practice Exam. Make sure that the person in charge of exam logistics has scheduled a preliminary walk-through with all of the CPX administrative staff. Although the responsibility for the CPX logistics should be in the hands of someone other than you, it is important that you coordinate with the chief administrator to be sure that all the needs of the SPs are understood and accounted for in the logistical plans. It is also helpful if you and the CPX administrator meet with all participating members of the administrative team (e.g., proctors, timer, video recordists, assistants) to make sure that everyone understands their individual responsibilities and has an opportunity to ask questions and try out what they will be rehearsing during the Practice Exam as preparation for their roles in the CPX.

CHAPTER ELEVEN

Training Options: Variations on the Training Sessions

Sometimes circumstances arise that necessitate rearranging the training of the skill sets or the focus within the various training sessions. The reasons for this shift usually revolve around the newness or complexity of the case in question, the experience of your SPs with standardized patient work, and your growing expertise as a coach.

Determining the SP Training Necessary

To determine how much and what type of training is necessary for your standardized patients, ask yourself these kinds of questions:

- How experienced are my SPs?
- Have any of the SPs performed this case or a similar one before?
- Does the fact that my SPs are actors or non-actors create any special circumstances?
- Does the case require performance of a strong emotion, a psychological or psychiatric condition (and consequently need more emphasis on portrayal)?
- How complicated is the checklist?
- Have the SPs ever been trained before to give feedback?
- How old are my SPs (very young or very old may require you to do more, or a different kind of, training)?

As you answer these questions, decide whether you need to compress or expand the sessions by length, number, or focus.

On the one hand, you might be able to reduce the number of sessions because you find yourself working with expert, rather than novice, SPs who have experience performing different kinds of cases in either teaching and/or assessment situations, or because one or another of them has already performed the case at another time.

On the other hand, if you are starting a new program, you might find yourself needing to increase the number of sessions because you are without one or another of the suggested resources, because the case is new or the SPs are new to acting, or because the SPs who are already actors are new to the standardization process. In other words, any time you determine that the required skills need to be configured differently than what has been described in the previous training sessions (in order to suit the situation or the SPs involved) means changing the training schedule. The following are examples of circumstances that might cause you to consider reorganizing the activities in one or more of the SPs' training sessions.

You Find Yourself Without a Specified Resource

You Have No Video Recordings

When you are training a new patient case, you will not have any video recordings because the case has not yet been performed. Of necessity, this will require you to do checklist training with your SPs in another manner. (See p. 247: When There Are No Video Recordings of the Case for Checklist Training.)

You Have No Assistant

You will have to rethink how to handle some of the training procedures if you do not have an assistant to interview the SPs when they are practicing the integration of all the skills, or when you need an assistant to help with the logistics during Training Session Four and the Practice Exam.

You or the SPs Feel the Need for Additional Training

When several complex tasks are combined in the same session, the learning must, of necessity, be split among the activities. Trying to train inexperienced SPs to learn multiple skills in the same session can be confusing and stressful for new SPs, as it can be for new coaches who often see so many things that need to be addressed that they may find it hard to know how best to handle all that is going on. If you find yourself in this situation, give each session a focus, a primary skill, to which you and the SPs can direct your attention and practice. This allows the SPs to perfect one part of their training before requiring them to learn another part, that is, to build their expertise one skill at a time.

For example, teaching the SPs how to give feedback in the form of written comments can be an intense process, particularly for new SPs who have never been trained to do this sort of thing before. This is one situation where you might consider holding a separate session for feedback only. You can do this separate session, similar to checklist training, by having the SPs watch a number of videos of performances. Following each viewing, the SPs would then fill out only the PPI portion of the checklist and practice writing comments in the from-the-patient's-perspective section. You can use video recordings of the same case that the SPs are going to perform if the feedback training is done within the context of a single case, but, in truth, the videos can be of any student/SP encounter because the PPI skills and the written feedback are generic communication skills that apply to any doctor–patient interaction. For this reason, you could consider combining feedback training for all the SPs from all the cases being trained for a given clinical skills examination into one session. This separate training session would still contain the elements described in chapter 9 (Training the SPs to Give Effective Written Feedback), but instead of building feedback training into Session Three, you could hold a separate feedback training session before any of the individual case training sessions begin—or at any other juncture that you think is appropriate during the various case training sessions (for example, before or after the checklist training session).

Another possibility is to double the number of sessions on a particular skill and shorten the length of each session. This strategy can work with any session, but, again, it is particularly effective with Training Session Three—the putting-it-all-together session. Doubling the number of sessions while shortening their length works particularly well when training complex geriatric cases with older SPs.

Here is how one actor new to standardized patient work put it:

> Being an SP is challenging work, which requires a different kind of improvisation where not only *the situation* is defined, but *what*-you-can-say-*when* is also specified. The challenge is to be able to do all of that and still have the performance appear spontaneous.... It takes time to get the hang of it.

Reorganizing the Middle Training Session Activities

If you determine that the SPs might need more performance training or that checklist training will have to be done at the same time that the SPs are continuing to perfect their portrayals—either because you have no video recordings or because you want to continue to strengthen the SPs' expertise in one or another of the skill areas—you can rearrange the middle sessions in a number of ways to accomplish your training goals. However, note that the first session must focus on orienting the SPs to the case training materials, the portrayal, and the simulated physical findings; and the final sessions must include clinician verification and the Practice Exam dress rehearsal.

When a Session Is Focused Solely on Portrayal

When you decide to focus a single training session on portrayal, try starting with these guidelines:

First, Do a Progressive Interview With all of the SPs

You can find a detailed description of this technique in Training Session One in chapter 7.

Next, Give Each SP the Opportunity to Perform the Complete Case With the Coach

Each SP will perform the case a minimum of two or three times while all of the *observing SPs* make notes on each other's performances. (The number of encounters you can do with each SP in a given session depends on the number of SPs you are training.)

Finally, Have the SPs Share Their Observations With Each Other After Each Practice Encounter

Then take time to compliment and adjust the SP's performance, going back into and repeating parts of the interaction as necessary. Remember the focus of this session is *performance*—that is, portrayal authenticity and accuracy of presentation. Therefore, everyone needs to be thoroughly familiar with the items on the checklist so that in the unfolding of their performances of the case, the SPs are not giving away checklist items. Consequently, the SPs must refer to the checklist and the guide to the checklist during performance training, even though they will not yet be required to fill out a checklist after each practice encounter.

Role Playing Is <u>Not</u> an Option in Training for High-Stakes Examinations

Portrayal, performance, checklist, and feedback coaching and practice are the responsibility of the SP coach. Therefore, even if you are short-handed, do *not* resort to having the SPs role play with each other as a substitute for not having an assistant coach or a clinician working with you. Instead, as previously described, have the observing SPs take notes while the coach is going through full encounters with each of them. Their notes (on what-happened-when and on anything the performing SP did that is different from their interpretation of the patient) can serve as reminders about performance issues and portrayal concerns the coach might want to go over with the SP with whom they just finished the encounter.

Having the SPs role play with each other can be a useful technique as part of SP training for performances in teaching situations. SP training for teaching purposes is, by its very nature, less intense and less demanding than training for high-stakes examinations. As such, it allows for the flexibility of letting the SPs role play their cases with one another in order to get a sense of the challenge the medical students are facing on their end of the interaction—which is not a bad experience to have.

However, in preparing SPs to perform in high-stakes examinations, role playing is not appropriate and should not be part of the training protocols. Because the SPs are trainees themselves, they do not understand the case from a coach's point of view, nor can they analyze the particular training needs of each SP in the way that the SP coach can and must do. In addition, the SPs were not hired for their skill in interviewing and taking medical histories, in performing the physical exam, or in any of the other clinical skills for which the SP coach's particular expertise is needed—expertise that allows the coach to determine which aspects of the case and which specific challenges he wants each SP to experience in each of the practice encounters.

When There Are No Video Recordings of the Case for Checklist Training

When the focus of a single training session is on checklist accuracy and no video recordings are available for this purpose, the SPs will be required to perform the cases as the basis for learning how to fill out the checklists. Therefore, if you do not have any videos, it is imperative that you focus on portrayal refinement in the session *prior to* checklist training. If you are confident in the SPs' portrayals of the case, all of you will be able to focus on the nuances of checklist training in a more concentrated way than if you are also concerned about the SPs having the facts accurately mem-orized, generating the right emotion at the right time, and/or producing an accurate simulation of the physical findings. Once all of the portrayal issues become second nature to the SPs, they can more readily concentrate on learning the nuances of recalling and recording observed behaviors on the checklist. Within reason, the more checklists the SPs have a chance to fill out and review, the better they will become at this important skill.

Repetition and review are the keys to checklist accuracy, as they are to all aspects of any kind of performance improvement.

As you can see, there are a number of possible variations for mixing and matching the diversity of skill sets that the SPs need to learn—including adjusting the number and length of training sessions required. Trust your instincts, then use your own good judgment to decide when and how to modify the training procedures. As always, let these finished performance criteria be your guide:

- 100% believability of the emotional aspects in the SPs' portrayals.
- Better than 90% overall accuracy of the SPs' presentations.
- Better than 85% overall accuracy rate of the SPs' checklists.
- Demonstrated expertise in the written feedback the SPs give to the students.

These are the measure of the collaborative efforts of everyone involved—you, your assistants, the administrative staff, and, of course, the SPs themselves. These are the ultimate fruits of the quality of the relationships you have established and of your work together with the SPs.

CHAPTER TWELVE

The Practice Exam: Final Dress Rehearsal

The Practice Exam is the final stage of preparation of the SPs for their performances in the actual administration of the CPX and, as such, is an integral part of the training protocols. It is the final dress rehearsal, completing the initial rehearsal phase begun in Training Session Four. The Practice Exam is a mock-up of an actual exam administration in which every SP for every case and all personnel—all staff, coaches, and SPs who will be involved in the actual clinical examination—are present to practice the exam logistics with residents (or other appropriate health care trainees) serving as the examinees. Think of the Practice Exam as a chance to fine tune both the SPs' performances and the logistical orchestration of the CPX event in a setting where finding mistakes becomes an opportunity to identify problems rather than a crisis to resolve in the midst of the actual testing of the medical students' clinical skills.

The Goal of the Practice Exam

By the end of the Practice Exam, the administrative staff should be able to expertly handle all aspects of the exam logistics. All SPs should be able to perform as indistinguishable from real patients in their portrayals, have better than a 90% overall accuracy rate in the content of their presentations (from facts to simulated physical findings), and be able within the exam timeframe to complete all the checklists with better than an 85% overall accuracy rate and give effective written feedback. All coaches should have been able to monitor at least one encounter of each SP they trained and give them feedback on both their performances and their checklist accuracy.

The Practice Exam Setting

The Practice Exam should take place in the actual or simulated clinic space where the CPX will be administered.

Summary of the Practice Exam Activities

During this final dress rehearsal, the chief administrator of the exam—as well as the timer (who is often the person giving instructions to the examinees and SPs over the intercom system), proctors, video recordist, and any assistants—will be running the Practice Exam as if it were the actual exam. The residents (examinees for the Practice Exam) will also need to be greeted, oriented, and debriefed. In fact, all activities during this Practice Exam session are the same as those in the actual clinical examination administrations—with one notable exception. During this Practice Exam administration, *all trained SPs for all of the cases will be present.* They will all rotate sequentially into their particular stations (the clinic exam room assigned to their case) so that each SP can go through at least two encounters with different residents to get a feel for the pacing of the exam and the rhythm of performing one encounter after another.

Reminders

There Should Be No Fewer Than 2 Days, but No More Than 1 Week Between the Practice Exam and the Start of the CPX

This break ensures that what the SPs have learned from the final dress rehearsal is fresh in their minds when they start performing in the CPX, and it also allows enough lead time to refine administrative procedures and to work with SPs or staff who were identified as having difficulties with their assignments during the Practice Exam.

Inform all of the SPs About the Performance Rotation Schedule for Their Particular Case

The rotation of all SPs, who have been trained in a given case, into and out of the station (exam room) assigned to their case is the one logistical feature that makes the Practice Exam different from an actual exam. As you know, during the actual CPX administrations, only *one* of the trained SPs from each of the cases will be present to perform their specific case. By contrast, during this Practice Exam, *all* of the SPs will be present to practice a few rounds of their case in this mock-up of the real exam. Therefore, in order for all of the SPs to get a feel for the rhythm and pacing of going from one encounter to another, a rotation system that is not disruptive to the examinees needs to be set up. Having an assistant available to handle the switching of the SPs into and out of their assigned clinic rooms after they have been through a minimum of two encounters is helpful on the day of the Practice Exam. (This assistant is not needed during an actual exam because there will be only one SP assigned to each station during the regular exam sessions.)

Here is how you might plan for and arrange the SPs' rotation schedule.

Number of SPs

If you are putting on an exam with two administrations per day, you will have trained three SPs for each case, a different SP to perform in each administration and the third as backup in the event that either of the other two SPs cannot make it to a scheduled performance. During this final rehearsal, all three SPs for all of the cases will be present. Therefore, if you are putting on an eight-station exam, there will be 24 SPs who, during this Practice Exam administration, need to be rotated into the eight clinic rooms where they will perform their cases.

Number of Examinees

Just as in an actual exam, there should be the same number of examinees scheduled to participate in the Practice Exam as there are stations in the exam. So, in an eight-station exam, there will be eight examinees moving from station to station until all of them have seen all of the cases.

Rotation Schedule

If this is the first time you are putting on a CPX, or if you have a number of new SPs or staff involved in the logistics of the exam, it is worth running the full number of encounters for the exam (eight encounters for an eight-station exam) during this final dress rehearsal, even though, from the SPs' training point of view, you would only need to run six encounters to give all three of the SPs the two-encounter, minimum amount of practice. So in the full Practice Exam scenario, you can split up the extra encounters in any way that seems appropriate. For example, if you wish to give certain SPs more practice, you can assign the two extra encounters in an eight-station exam to those SPs. Even though it is easiest if all the SPs rotate into and out of their stations at the same time, if you have an assistant managing the SP rotations, you can stagger the "ins and outs" in any way you see fit.

All of the SPs portraying patient cases requiring a physical examination should be gowned for the whole of the Practice Exam. While one of the three SPs is in the exam room performing, another is watching the encounter from the monitoring room and filling out a checklist at the end of the encounter along with the performing SP. The third SP is in line ready to move into the station when it is time to do so. At the switching point, the in-line SP moves into the clinic room, the performing SP moves into the monitoring room, the monitoring room SP moves to the in-line position—while the exam continues without a break in continuity.

The Practice Exam Activities (Time Varies by Number of Cases)

Unlike the four previous case-specific training sessions, the Practice Exam brings together the three essential groups of people who will participate in the CPX, but who have not yet worked together as an integrated unit. These groups include all the SPs and their coaches; the examinees and those who will orient them before the exam and debrief them after they have seen all of the patients; and the administrative support staff who need to practice doing their jobs, which includes communicating with the SPs, the examinees, and each other.

Intermittent Monitoring and Feedback to Maintain SP Accuracy

Intermittently monitoring and regularly giving feedback to the SPs on both their performances and checklists is the most efficient way to maintain consistently high levels of SP accuracy.

As mentioned in Training Session Four (see chapter 10), the reason for intermittent monitoring of SP performances throughout each exam administration is to help the SPs maintain the high standards they have achieved during training. The natural tendency when performing the same case for an extended period of time is for the SPs' performances to drift and their concentration to waiver, which affect their performance and checklist accuracy. Research has shown that coaches can help SPs maintain error-free performances and a high degree of checklist accuracy throughout the entire examination if the coaches themselves randomly monitor their SPs' performances and fill out checklists during the encounter (Wallace et al., 1999).

Ongoing feedback on performance and comparison of checklists should be done with all the SPs who have been monitored. This is best done at the break and at the end of each exam administration. Do not try to give feedback to the SPs after each encounter. This can disrupt the exam logistics, and popping in and out between every encounter to let the SP know what he is doing wrong can have a negative psychological effect on him. This technique for maintaining high levels of accuracy should, of course, be initiated by the coaches during the Practice Exam.

If the SPs see their relationship with their coach as a partnership, they will look forward to being observed because they know they have a distinct forum in which to

- discuss concerns about the unique ways a medical student approached an aspect of the case.
- ask questions they have about how to record on the checklist a student's atypical behavior.

Note: *To accomplish this critical task of randomly monitoring equal numbers of SP encounters, coaches cannot be responsible for any other activities during CPX testing, namely, any administrative responsibilities for the day-to-day running of the exam.*

Other Measures to Ensure Consistently High SP Accuracy

Besides intermittently monitoring and giving feedback to the SPs on their performances and checklists, being aware of the other elements that ensure dependably high accuracy is the first step toward achieving that goal. Here are a few to consider:

Checklist Length

Generally speaking, the fewer the number of checklist items, the higher the SP accuracy; the higher the number of items, the lower the accuracy (Colliver & Williams, 1993). Experience in the California Consortium for the Assessment of Clinical Competence has shown that a combined total of 25 to 30 uncomplicated history, physical examination, and information-sharing items is the maximum allowable per checklist in order to ensure—and reasonably expect—that the SPs will perform at or above the 85% overall accuracy rate.

Amount of Time Allotted for Checklist Completion

Clarity of the Language Used in the Checklist

Quality of the Information in the Guide to the Checklist

Habitual Use of the Guide as a Reference by the SPs Whenever They Are Determining How to Record Examinee Behavior

Scheduled Breaks for the SPs During the Exam to Counteract the Fatigue Factor

The longer an SP performs, the more chances there are for errors, particularly in recording examinee behaviors on the checklist. It is a well-known self-reported phenomenon that after performing with the first few examinees, what happens in subsequent encounters tends to blend together in the SP's mind with what happened in previous encounters. Therefore, all else being equal, the more encounters an SP is required to do in a given day, the greater is the likelihood for inaccuracies in their successive checklists, unless certain measures such as the following are taken to prevent and reduce fatigue:

- Schedule the SPs to perform for no more than 6 hours on any given day.
- Encourage the SPs to renew their concentration consistently at the beginning of each encounter. Although this is easier said than done, a conscious effort to treat each new encounter as if it were the first does seem to help the SPs stay sharper in their performances and more accurate in filling out the checklists.
- Schedule breaks during any exam administration that has more than six encounters or that runs longer than 3 hours.

In addition to diminishing the effects of the fatigue factor, scheduling breaks in the middle of their performances using the guidelines just mentioned helps to physically and psychologically separate the previous part of the exam from the next part—in essence giving the SPs a fresh start.

Orientation and Debriefing of Examinees

Anyone taking a high-stakes performance exam is anxious. Therefore, anything reasonable that can be done to allay the examinees' fears is worth doing, so that their performances represent their highest skill level. Sending out clearly written guidelines before the exam helps, as does an orientation session on the day of testing during which the examinees have a chance to ask and get answers to their questions. This, of course, applies equally to the residents participating in the Practice Exam and the medical students taking the CPX. At a minimum, orientation and debriefing should include the following:

Orientation

Orientation should include such information as the kinds of skills being assessed; the number of stations; examinee start stations; the timing of encounters and interstation exercises (write-ups); exam procedures and announcements; the way the examinees should handle the intimate exams (breast, pelvic, genital, and rectal exams); the generic content of the interstation write-ups; a reminder that the examinees' performances will be video recorded; and the number and timing of breaks.

Debriefing

Debriefing should include giving the examinees such information as how the exam will be scored, what will be included in the score reports they will receive, when the examinees will get those results, and so on. Debriefing can also provide an opportunity for the examinees to discuss how they feel about the experience they just had.

It is preferable for a faculty member familiar with the exam to do both the orientation and the debriefing, although this is not always possible. Often it is the director of the standardized patient program who interacts with the examinees at the beginning and the end of the CPX. However, no matter who does the orientation and particularly the debriefing, they must be careful not to discuss details of the cases with the examinees in order to protect the security and integrity of the exam.

Announcements

Although it might seem like a small matter, the language used to communicate publicly with the SPs and the examinees sets a tone for their exam experience. The goal is to make the environment as supportive as possible while still being professional. How the chief proctor and other administrative staff communicate with each other and with the SPs also affects the atmosphere in which the examinees are participating.

Announcements are the formal verbal directives that the timer will give the examinees for starting the exam, entering and exiting the clinic stations, taking a break, warning how much time is left on a given activity, and so on. The announcements should be clear, respectful, and short (to not unduly disrupt the activity the examinee is engaged in). Here are examples of several types of announcements you will need to make:

- "You may read the presenting situation (station instructions)— then enter the room when you are ready."
- "You have 5 minutes left."
- "You may move on to the next station."
- "Student doctor, you're needed in the hallway" (as a means of letting the student know that it is time to end the encounter and start the interstation exercise).

In addition to rehearsing announcements to guide the examinees through the process during the Practice Exam, the exam administrator, proctors, and timer need to rehearse their communications with each other and with the examinees and the SPs. Depending on the kind of data collection system you use, the timer might also need to independently coordinate with a video recordist. For these kinds of communications, walkie-talkies with headsets work best because they allow all of the staff to interact and simultaneously hear each other without interfering with what the examinees and SPs are doing.

Preparation of the SPs for the Actual Exam

As the coach, even if you gave the SPs a preview of the upcoming CPX during Training Session Four, it is a good idea (after you have debriefed the Practice Exam with the SPs) to go over guidelines for the CPX with them once again.

Review of CPX Guidelines

- Review the exam performance schedule, expectations you have about pre- and postexam SP arrival and departure, parking arrangements, and any other relevant administrative matters.

- Remind the SPs about the practical and psychological preparation they need to do before each performance. For example, discuss arriving early enough to change into patient gowns, create any make-up/moulage, and check their assigned exam room to make sure it is set up properly. Then, after accomplishing all of these practical tasks, the SPs should allow ample time to get into character before the start of the exam.

- Discuss any exam situations the SPs will encounter that were not part of training. Dealing with *down stations* is one example. When an exam administration does not have a full complement of examinees, an open slot (which would have been taken up by the missing examinee) will rotate through the stations. The SPs will need to know when that open slot, or down station, is at their room so that they know they will not be performing during that particular encounter. They will also need to know whether or not you want them to remain in the room or if they can relax in the SP break room once the examinees are out of the hallway and engaged in the encounter in the other rooms.

- Remind the SPs to notify you or your assistant, as soon as possible, if they are unable to perform as scheduled.

Other Considerations When Preparing the SPs for the CPX

Debriefing the SPs After Every Administration

We need to be sure that the SPs have come "out of character" after they have completed their performances so that they can safely leave for the day. This is particularly true for SPs who have been performing cases that have strong emotional components to them, such as depression, anxiety over bad news, anger—to name a few. Most actors are aware of the need to release the feelings that might have built up in them personally as a result of performing the case repeatedly. However, it is still a good idea to check in with the SPs—actors and non-actors alike—to find out how they are doing.

Sometimes the SPs are not aware that they are carrying the patient's emotion until they start talking with you. So keeping them around for a few extra minutes is worthwhile, even if they seem all right. Just chatting with them and listening to their stories about their CPX experiences is often all it takes for them to shake their unconsciously held feelings.

In addition, when talking with them about their experiences, we can learn how the cases are working from the SPs' point of view. Firsthand data from the very people who are performing the cases provide us with information that can substantially help improve the case materials for future use.

Arranging Supplies and Equipment

The exam rooms should be fully outfitted with all the supplies and equipment usually found in primary care clinics. (If the rooms are equipped with only what is needed for each station, there is a risk of cueing students to particular aspects of the physical exam required by a specific case.)

All rooms should have an ample supply of linens (gowns, sheets, pillows, pillow cases, and blankets) available for use from the first training session through the last administration of the CPX.

The Coach's Preparation for the CPX and Examination Follow-up Activities

Your preparation for the CPX is similar to the preparation you did for the Practice Exam, with the most significant exception being that only one SP per case will be scheduled for each CPX administration. The other aspects of the CPX, which you may or may not be involved in, are the follow-up activities related to how the medical students performed on the exam. Whether or not you are involved in any of these activities, it is worth knowing what they consist of so that you have a sense of how your part fits into the whole clinical assessment process.

The primary activities following the CPX have to do with scoring and analysis of individual and collective data from the checklists. From this information, the CPX advisory committee can determine pass/fail cuts and honors, and which medical students need clinical skills remediation. In addition, based on class performance, faculty can decide which parts of the curriculum might need attention. Letters to the students along with their score reports need to be prepared and delivered to them in a timely fashion. Remediation activities, including a retake of the CPX, need to be designed, scheduled, and carried out.

Throughout the Practice Exam, you have had a chance to monitor your SPs as each of them performed with different examinees. You have also been able to compare the checklists you filled out during their clinical encounters with the ones the SPs submitted right after each interaction. So now, at the end of the Practice Exam, you are able to debrief with the SPs about your observations and their experiences before they start working with the medical students in the upcoming actual examination. This is a good opportunity to tie up loose ends in the SPs' performances, find out how they are feeling about things in general, congratulate them on all of their hard work, and cheer them on to the experience they are about to have with the students they have been training so hard to work with.

What you have done to prepare your SPs for this work is a tremendous accomplishment—and one that should make you proud of yourself and the role you are playing in helping the medical school faculty help their students achieve excellence in their clinical skills. Congratulate yourself and really take in the compliments that the SPs are sure to give you as a result of the excellent, hard work that all of you have done together.

Afterword

So here you are. You have meticulously worked through all this training, your SPs and you have put on multiple administrations of the CPX, you have collected and had the data analyzed, and the score reports have been sent out along with the SPs' written feedback to the students. Now let's reflect on the significance of what you have done—the significance of what we are all doing. As SP coaches and educators, we are responsible for two of the standards by which our medical students' clinical skills are being judged: the authenticity and accuracy of the *standardized patients'* performances and the accuracy of the data that the SPs are recording on the *students'* performances. The accuracy of the SPs in accomplishing these tasks depends on how well we have selected the SPs, on the quality of our coaching, and on another important factor that is in our hands as SP coaches and in the hands of the case author(s) who design the checklist and create the items; namely, making sure that the wording of each checklist item and the intent behind that item is clear. When these criteria are met, the responsibility for the accuracy of the data collected is then wholly dependent on the SPs' portrayals and on their checklist completion. "Well, that's a given," you might say. It is a given, only if we, as SP coaches, care enough about this accuracy, are diligent enough in training, and rigorous enough in monitoring our SPs' portrayals and checklist performances to know for sure how accurate the data are that are being collected. "If the data that the psychometrician receives is flawed, no psychometric technique can overcome the errors in the data" (E. R. Petrusa, personal communication, February 6, 2006).

What we are coaching our SPs to do is no small matter. In fact, it is very significant. The foundation for the interpretation of the data and the consequences for the students that result from any high-stakes performance exam rest with the SPs because it is they who provide the primary data on which everything else depends. Therefore, as E. R. Petrusa, a medical

educator whose research has contributed to the growth in understanding of the psychometric qualities of SP-based examinations, has stated,
"If that foundation is not solid, everything built on it is flawed." Those
flaws in portrayal and those errors on the checklists whether against the
students or in their favor

> have huge consequences for people's lives. In high-stakes ex-
> ams, careers are on the line: a student might be delayed from
> getting into residency training; may not be licensed to practice
> medicine; may have to spend another year in medical school
> with substantial financial consequences. Or students and fac-
> ulty may go forward, thinking students who pass the CPX
> are competent because of the trust they have in the SPs as the
> primary data providers [and I would add *and the trust they
> have in the SP coaches who have selected and trained them*].
> However, if those pass decisions come from error-prone data,
> that sense of confidence is unfounded and has implications for
> future patient care. (E. R. Petrusa, personal communication,
> February 6, 2006)

As we know, in other performance-based areas of professional study—
such as music, film directing, sports such as figure skating, and law—the
candidate's abilities are judged by a jury of experts from the particular specialty involved. These experts are the holders of the standards of quality in
their field, but in medicine—because of the intrinsic situation that makes
it difficult for clinical faculty to directly observe medical students often
enough to produce a fair and reliable measure of the student's abilities—
standardized patients have become the surrogates for those direct faculty
observations. This is why SP coaches must maintain the highest levels of
quality all of the time in every aspect of SP training and performances.

The bottom line is that everyone assumes that the data derived from
the checklists are accurate. But the truth is that unless the SPs' performances are regularly monitored, no one will know for sure how accurate
the data are—not the SPs, not the coaches, not the faculty, not the psy-
chometricians. Why? Because the data from these SP-based examinations
in and of themselves do not indicate the accuracy of the SPs' recall or
the correctness of the SPs' judgments when they fill out the checklists.
Unless we make extraordinary efforts to train our SPs well and monitor
their performances throughout all of the administrations of the CPX, we
will be collecting data and we will be reporting data, but we will not
know how accurate those data really are. We will not know what errors
are being made. We will not know if those errors are ones the students
are making in their performances or are ones the SPs are making in their

recall or interpretation of the checklist items. This is an interesting facet of the complexity of what we are doing—and of the uniqueness of these standardized patient performance examinations.

Unless someone, who understands the case and knows the criteria by which each item on the checklist is to be assessed, sits down and fills out checklists while watching the videos, then compares those checklists with those the SPs have filled out, no one can tell how accurate each checklist is. (And practically no one does this except the coaches because it is so labor intensive.) The point I hope I have made is that it is the SP educators, the SP coaches, who hold the standard. The truth is that we are the ones who are accountable for the baseline quality assurance of the data collected during these clinical skills assessments.

It is my hope that the principles and procedures I have presented in this book will become part of the continuing dialogue on standardized patient training that has already started among us. It is this dialogue that inspires us to question what we are doing, to hold ourselves accountable to the highest standards of excellence, to explore ways to collectively improve and assure the quality of our SPs' work, to maintain our integrity, and to deeply value ourselves and the work that we are doing. We must never forget that we are an integral, significant part of our medical students' training and always remember that our SPs and we, as their coaches, are key participants in the assessment of the clinical competence of each new generation of physicians.

References

Adler, S. (1988). *The technique of acting*. New York: Bantam.

The American Heritage College Dictionary (3rd ed.). (1997). New York: Houghton Mifflin.

Association of American Medical Colleges. (1999, October). *Contemporary issues in medicine: Communication in medicine* (Report III, Medical School Objectives Project). Washington, DC: Association of American Medical Colleges.

Barrows, H. S. (1999). *Training standardized patients to have physical findings*. Springfield: Southern Illinois University School of Medicine.

Bayer Institute for Health Care Communication. (2003). *Clinician-patient communication to enhance health outcomes* (Workbook; Rev. ed.). West Haven, CT: Bayer Institute.

Bickley, L. S., & Szilagyi, P. G. (2003). *Bates' guide to physical examination and history taking* (8th ed.). Philadelphia: Lippincott Williams & Wilkins.

Brook, P. (1968). *The empty space*. London: MacGibbon & Kee.

Bruder, M., Cohn, L. M., Olnek, M., Pollack, N., Previto, R., & Zigler, S. (1986). *A practical handbook for the actor*. New York: Vintage.

Cohen, R. (1978). *Acting power: An introduction to acting*. Palo Alto, CA: Mayfield.

Cole, T., & Chinoy, H. K. (Eds.). (1986). *Directors on directing: A source book of the modern theatre* (Rev. ed.). New York & London: Macmillan.

Colliver, J. A., & Williams, R. G. (1993, June). Technical issues: Test application. *Academic Medicine, 68*(6), 454–460.

Cottrell, J. (1975). *Laurence Olivier*. London: Weidenfeld & Nicolson.

De Champlain, A. F., Margolis, M. J., King, A., & Klass, D. J. (1997, October). Standardized patients' accuracy in recording examinees' behaviors using checklists. *Academic Medicine, 72*(10), Supplement 1, S85–S87.

Essential elements of communication in medical encounters: The Kalamazoo Consensus Statement. (2001, April). *Academic Medicine, 76*(4), 390–393.

Funke, L., & Booth, J. E. (1961). *Actors Talk About Acting*. Random House: New York.

Geldard, R. G. (2000). *Ancient Greece: A guide to sacred places.* Wheaton, IL: Quest Books.

Heine, N., Garman, K., Wallace, P., Bartos, R., & Richards, A. (2003). An analysis of standardized patient checklist errors and their effect on student scores. *Medical Education, 37,* 99–104.

Huber, P., Baroffio, A., Chamot, E., Herrmann, F., Nendaz, M. R., & Vu, N.V. (2005). Effects of item and rater characteristics on checklist recording: What should we look for? *Medical Education, 39,* 852–858.

Hunt, G. (1977). *How to audition: Advice from a casting director.* New York: Harper & Row.

Kraytman, M. (1991). *The complete patient history* (2nd ed.). New York: McGraw-Hill, Health Professions Division.

Macy, W. H. (2004, October 24). *Inside the Actors Studio.* Interview with James Lipton, [Television broadcast]. Los Angeles: Bravo TV.

Mamet, D. (1997). *True and false: Heresy and common sense for the actor.* New York: Pantheon.

Meisner, S., & Longwell, D. (1987). *Sanford Meisner on acting.* New York: Vintage.

Mink, O., Owen, K. Q., & Mink, B. P. (1993). *Developing high performance people: The art of coaching.* Cambridge, MA: Perseus.

Orient, J. M., & Sapira, J. D. (2005). *Sapira's art and science of bedside diagnosis.* Philadelphia: Lippincott, Williams, & Wilkins.

Petrusa, E. R. (2002). Clinical performance assessments. In G. R. Norman, C. P. M. Van der Vleuten, & D. I. Newble, (Eds.), *International handbook of research in medical education* (pp. 673–709). Dordrecht, The Netherlands: Kluwer Academic.

Seidel, H. M., Ball, J. W., Dains, J. E., Benedict, G. W. (2003). *Mosby's guide to physical examination* (5th ed.). St. Louis: Mosby.

Shapiro, M. (1998). *The director's companion.* Fort Worth, TX: Harcourt Brace.

Shurtleff, M. (1978). *Audition: Everything an actor needs to know to get the part.* New York: Walker.

Stanislavsky, C. (1958/1999). *Stanislavky's legacy: A collection of comments on a variety of aspects of an actor's life.* (E. Reynolds Hapgood, Trans.). New York: Routledge/A Theatre Arts Book (Original work published, 1958).

Swartz, M. H. (2002). *Textbook of physical diagnosis: History and examination* (4th ed.) Philadelphia: Saunders.

Tamblyn, R. M., Grad, R., Gayton, D., Petrella, L., Reid, T., & McGill Drug Utilization Research Group. (1997). Impact of inaccuracies in standardized patient portrayal and reporting on physician performance during blinded clinic visits. *Teaching and Learning in Medicine, 9*(1), 25–28.

Tamblyn, R. M., Klass, D. J., Schnabl, G. K., & Kopelow. M. L. (1991). The accuracy of standardized patient presentation. *Medical Education, 25,* 100–109.

Vu, N. V., & Barrows, H. S. (1994). Use of standardized patients in clinical assessments: Recent developments and measurement findings. *Educational Researcher, 23*(3), 23–30.

Vu, N. V., Marcy, M. M., Colliver, J. A., Verhulst, S. J., Travis, T. A., & Barrows, H. S. (1992). Standardized (simulated) patients' accuracy in recording clinical performance checklist items. *Medical Education, 26*, 99–104.

Wallace, P. A., Heine, N. J., Garman, K. A., Bartos, R., & Richards, A. (1999). Effect of varying amounts of feedback on standardized patient checklist accuracy in clinical practice examinations. *Teaching and Learning in Medicine, 11*, 148–152.

Weston, J. (1996). *Directing actors: Creating memorable performances for film and television.* Studio City, CA: Michael Wiese Productions.

White, M. K., & Bonvicini, K. (2003). *The annotated bibliography for clinician patient communication to enhance health outcomes.* Annotated bibliographies. Retrieved July 14, 2006, from: www.healthcarecomm.com.

Additional Readings on Acting and Directing

Adler, S. (1988). *The technique of acting.* New York: Bantam.

Bates, B. (1987). *The way of the actor: A path to knowledge and power.* Boston: Shambala.

Brook, P. (1968). *The empty space.* London: MacGibbon & Kee.

Bruder, M., Cohn, L. M., Olnek, M., Pollack, N., Previto, R., & Zigler, S. (1986). *A practical handbook for the actor.* New York: Vintage.

Chekhov, M. (1991). *On the technique of acting.* New York: HarperCollins.

Clurman, H. (1997). *On directing.* New York: Fireside.

Cohen, R. (1978). *Acting power: An introduction to acting.* Palo Alto, CA: Mayfield.

Hagen, U. (with Frankel, H.). (1973). *Respect for acting.* New York: Macmillan.

Mamet, D. (1991). *On directing film.* New York: Penguin Books.

Manley, B. (1998). *My breath in art: Acting from within.* New York: Applause Books.

Meisner, S., & Longwell, D. (1987). *Sanford Meisner on acting.* New York: Vintage.

Sherman, E. (1976). *Directing the film: Film directors on their art.* Boston: Little, Brown.

Spolin, V. (1983). *Improvisation for the theater: A handbook of teaching and directing techniques.* Evanston, IL: Northwestern University Press.

Stanislavsky, C. (1946). *An actor prepares.* (E. Reynolds Hapgood, Trans.). New York: Theatre Arts (Original work published 1936).

Stanislavsky, C. (1948). *My life in art.* New York: Theatre Arts Books.

Stanislavsky, C. (1962). *Building a character.* (E. Reynolds Hapgood, Trans.). New York: Theatre Arts Books (Original work published 1949).

Stanislavsky, C. (1980). *Creating a role.* (E. Reynolds Hapgood, Trans.). New York: Theatre Arts Books (Original work published 1961).

Stanislavsky, C. (1999). *Stanislavky's legacy: A collection of comments on a variety of aspects of an actor's life* (E. Reynolds Hapgood, Trans.). New York: Routledge/Theatre Arts Book (Original work published 1958).

Strasberg, L. (1988). *A dream of passion: The development of The Method*. New York: Penguin Books.

Wangh, S. (2000). *An acrobat of the heart: A physical approach to acting inspired by the work of Jerzy Grotowski*. New York: Random House/Vintage.

APPENDIX A

Maria Gomez
Case Materials

Demographic Form

Maria Gomez

PRESENTING SYMPTOMS: Lower abdominal pain for past 2 days

ACTUAL DIAGNOSIS: Urinary tract infection (UTI)

DIFFERENTIAL DIAGNOSIS: Pelvic inflammatory disease (PID)–
chlamydia, gonorrhea
Ectopic pregnancy
Cervicitis
Vaginitis
Gastroenteritis
Sexually transmitted disease (STD)–
trichomonas, chlamydia
Pyelonephritis
Kidney stone
Urinary tract infection

CLINICAL CONSULTANT: Stacie J. O. San Miguel, MD

CASE AUTHORS: Peggy Wallace, PhD
University of California, San Diego
Stacie J. O. San Miguel, MD
University of California, San Diego
Anita J. Richards
University of California, San Diego

PATIENT NAME: Maria Gomez

PATIENT DEMOGRAPHICS:

Age: 21 years old
Sex: Female
Race: Latina
Height: Average
Weight: Average

MATERIALS and EQUIPMENT NEEDED:
Pelvic/rectal exam results in folder.

Pelvic Examination Results
External genitalia: no redness of the skin or lesions.
Vagina: slight white discharge in the vaginal vault; no fishy odor.
Cervix: no discharge; no cervical motion tenderness.
Uterus: mild fundal tenderness with palpation; no masses felt.
Adnexa: no masses or tenderness.

Rectal Examination Results
The anus appears normal on inspection.
On digital examination, there is normal sphincter tone.
Small amount of brown stool in the rectal vault that is heme negative.
No masses found.

PROFILE:
Maria Gomez is a 21-year-old Latina who has come to the doctor's office because of stomach pains that she has been experiencing for the past 2 days. A friend told her it might be a bladder infection. She is a college student starting work on her master's degree. She lives at home and is still covered by her parents' health insurance. She does not want her parents to know that she is sexually active or, if it comes up in the encounter, that she might be pregnant, or even to know that she is dating the boyfriend they disapproved of because he is neither Latino nor Catholic.

EVALUATION OBJECTIVES:

1. Elicit an accurate and relevant medical history based on the patient's symptoms, including the risk factors for the problems in the differential listed earlier and for recurrent infections.
2. Demonstrate a knowledge of the appropriate physical examination components that will help confirm a diagnosis.
3. Elicit cultural and religious beliefs that create the patient's unique perspective.
4. Establish trust by showing interest, curiosity, and openness to the patient's concerns and beliefs.
5. Discover how the patient understands her illness (the patient's perspective).
6. Demonstrate understanding of the patient's perspective. (Empathic listening.)
7. Detect verbal and nonverbal cues that indicate that the patient is worried/concerned.

8. Demonstrate, by the tone of the student's action (verbal/nonverbal), a genuine concern for the patient's total well-being. (Address the patient's feelings.)
9. Demonstrate an ability to share information with the patient in a way that the patient can understand and is respectful of her point of view.
10. Work toward a plan that takes into consideration both the student's assessment and treatment plan (student's perspective) as well as the patient's concerns about her symptoms, follow-up care, and confidentiality (patient's perspective).

Presenting Situation
and
Instructions to the Student

Maria Gomez

Maria Gomez is a 21-year-old female who has come to the primary care clinic where you work complaining of stomach pains. She has been experiencing these pains for the past 2 days.

Vital signs:

Temperature:	98.9°
Pulse:	78
Respiration:	12
Blood pressure:	105/60

You are to

- take a relevant history.
- perform an appropriate physical exam.
- tell the patient what you believe is going on with her and discuss the next steps in her care.

You will have **20 minutes** to perform these tasks.

You will hear an announcement over the intercom when there are **5 minutes** remaining in the encounter.

At the **end of the encounter,** you will hear, "Student doctor, you are needed in the hallway."

You will then have **10 minutes** to write an assessment and plan on this patient outside the patient room.

Training Materials

Maria Gomez

CASE SUMMARY

Maria Gomez is a 21-year-old Latina who has come to the doctor's office because of stomach pains that she has been experiencing for the past 2 days. A friend told her it might be a bladder infection. She is a college student starting work on her master's degree. She lives at home and is still covered by her parents' health insurance. She does not want her parents to know that she is sexually active or, if it comes up in the encounter, that she might be pregnant, or even to know that she is still dating the boyfriend they disapproved of because he is neither Latino nor Catholic.

Your challenge as the standardized patient is threefold:

1. To appropriately and accurately respond to questions about Maria Gomez's symptoms and medical history while faithfully reproducing the pain during the physical exam and the emotions Maria feels if the student convinces her she might be pregnant.
2. To observe the student's behavior while you are performing the case.
3. To accurately recall the student's behavior and complete the performance checklist which will partially determine the student's grade on this clinical skills examination.

PRESENTATION/EMOTIONAL TONE

Maria is a pleasant young woman; however, she is shy and guarded when talking about her sex life. She will answer the doctor's questions but is embarrassed if asked to elaborate with details. In other words, the doctor has to "help" her talk about her sexual activities. She is most comfortable if the student doctor just asks her questions to which she can simply give one-word answers.

Dress

You are in a gown sitting on the side of the exam table when the medical student walks in. You do not wear much make-up or jewelry. You have on simple earrings, a silver crucifix around your neck, and a watch.

Reason for Clinic Visit

When the student asks what brings you in to the clinic today, you respond:

> "I've had this crampy pain in the middle of my stomach for the last 2 days. I noticed it right here (gesture with the flat palm of your hand in the middle lower abdominal area when you say this) when I woke up a couple of days ago."

If the student asks you if you have any idea what might be wrong, you can say,

> "One of my friends thought I might have a bladder infection. She said she had a similar kind of pain and that's what it was. So...."

Changes in Demeanor During the Encounter

At the beginning of the encounter, you think you might have a bladder infection because that's what your friend, who had similar pain, was diagnosed with. However, during the course of the interview, you become fearful and anxious if the student doctor convinces you that (despite the birth control measures you've taken) you need to have a pregnancy test— or other tests to rule out sexually transmitted diseases. In addition to what these possibilities could mean for your future, you are worried that your parents will find out that you are sexually active.

HISTORY OF PRESENT ILLNESS

When you woke up a couple days ago the pain was mild. But it has not gone away since you first noticed it. In fact, it has gotten slightly worse.

Pain Symptoms

- **Location** – In the middle lower abdomen above the pubic bone. It's in the same place it started. It covers the full area of your hand.
- **Description** – Feels "crampy."
- **Constant/intermittent** – Has been constant since it started.
- **Better or worse** – Nothing makes the pain better or worse. In other words, it's not any better if you're sitting, standing, or lying down. The pain does NOT change (get better or worse) after eating, urinating, or having a bowel movement.

  If the student ONLY asks you if the pain *has gotten* better or worse *since it started* (2 days ago), your answer is **"Yes, it has gotten worse."** However, this is not the same as Item #4 on the checklist. (See Guide to the Checklist.)

  You have NOT taken any medications for the pain.

- **Intensity** – On a scale of 1 to 10 with "1" being a barely noticeable pain and "10" being the worst pain you've ever experienced, *this abdominal pain started out a "2" two days ago and has increased to about a "4" now.*

    Do NOT describe the intensity of your pain in "numbers" unless the student gives you a scale to choose from. Otherwise, just tell the student, **"It's bad, but not too bad."**

- **Radiation** – The pain does NOT go anywhere else.

- **Other pain questions**

    Any other questions about the pain, you answer in the negative. For example, the pain:

    – Does NOT wake you up at night.

    – Does NOT interfere with your normal activities.

Other Symptoms
The student may ask you if you've experienced any of the following:

- **Nausea/vomiting** – None

- **Changes in eating habits** – None

    You have been able to eat normally for the past 2 days. You had nothing unusual to eat the night before you woke up with the pain.

    (Trying to remember what you had to eat) **"I think I had a cheese pizza and a salad with a diet coke. That's usually what I have after I finish studying."**

- **Fever** – **"Not that I've noticed."**

- **Changes in bowel habits** – No changes. Normal formed brown stool once a day in the morning.

- **Blood in urine** – You haven't noticed any blood.

- **Increase in urinary frequency** – You notice that you *are* having to "go to the bathroom" more frequently. If asked about urinary frequency, tell the student:

    "Yes, I am having to go a lot more often. It seems like I have to go every hour or two."

    You get up to urinate at night on the same schedule.

- **Urgency** – You have a strong urge to go the bathroom.

    "When I feel the need to go, I have to go right away."

- **Amount of urine** – Over the past 2 days, because you go to the bathroom so frequently, there often isn't very much urine when you actually try to urinate.

- **Vaginal burning OR pain/burning on urination** – **"Yes—for about 3 days now."** (The pain is associated with burning.)

- **Vaginal discharge** – You are embarrassed to talk about this. If the student simply asks if you are having a vaginal discharge, you only say, **"Yes, I am."**

Wait for the student to ask for details about the vaginal discharge. Then give as much information as you feel comfortable giving, appropriate to the question.

– The discharge is white.
– You have discharge a lot of the time, but it seems as if you're having more the past couple of days.
– You are now using a panty liner to keep your underwear clean. *You change the panty liner two or three times a day.*
– There is *no odor* to the discharge; that is, it is not foul-smelling.

- **Vaginal bleeding** – Not in the past 2 days. Only when you're having your period.
- **Vaginal itching** – None
- **Pain with intercourse** – (If the student hasn't found out that you have a boyfriend and are sexually active, hesitate, look a little embarrassed and concerned, then nod and say: "I *am* having some pain." (The pain with intercourse has been only in the past 2 days.)

PAST MEDICAL HISTORY
Overall Health
You describe yourself as being a very healthy person. You only get an occasional cold and have never had any major illnesses.

You have NO HISTORY of urinary tract infections.
You have NEVER experienced anything like this before.

Previous Illnesses/Injuries
None

Allergies
None

Past Hospitalizations
You have never been hospitalized or had any surgeries of any kind.

MEDICATIONS
Prescription drugs – Depoprovera
You have been on Depoprovera for the past 6 months as a means of birth control.

Over the counter (OTC) drugs – Tylenol occasionally for headaches.
Illicit/street drugs – None

MENSTRUAL HISTORY
You are not comfortable talking about this subject or about Depoprovera; therefore, you only answer whatever the student asks. For example, When was your last menstrual period? **"Two months ago."** Are your periods

irregular? **"They have been lately."** How long have they been irregular? **"Since about 6 months ago."** Did anything happen 6 months ago that caused them to become irregular? **"I started Depoprovera."** OR Are you worried about your irregularity? **"No, not really."** [See Dealing with Open-Ended Questions and Guidelines for Disclosure on the last page of these Training Materials.]

- You started menstruating when you were 12 years old.
- **Your periods:**
  Before 6 months ago, your periods were normal (moderate flow every 28 days for 5 days). Since you started *Depoprovera* 6 months ago, your periods have been irregular.
- **What you have been told about Depoprovera:**
  1. Your periods can be irregular while you are on Depoprovera—and your periods might even stop altogether.
  2. That you would be protected from getting pregnant if:
     – you got your first shot within 5 days of the beginning of your last menstrual period (which you did).
     – you got your shots every 12 weeks (which you are doing).
  3. That Depoprovera is 98% effective in preventing pregnancy (which is the same as birth control pills). You decided on this method because it's easier to remember and your parents wouldn't find out.
  4. That the way Depoprovera stops pregnancy is by keeping you from ovulating—so there is no egg available to fertilize.
  5. That you might experience weight gain, nausea, breast tenderness, headaches.
     You've experienced none of these side effects.
- **Birth control**
  Here's a summary of your birth control history:
  1. Before you started dating your present boyfriend (Chris), you were never sexually active.
  2. Eight months ago you started dating Chris.
  3. Seven months ago you started having sexual intercourse (without any protection except for condoms "most of the time").
  4. Six months ago you got scared and went to Planned Parenthood to start birth control shots.
  5. You are supposed to get *a shot every 3 months.*
  6. You have had *2 shots so far (6 months ago and 3 months ago).* You are due for another shot next week.
  7. You decided on Depoprovera so that your mother wouldn't find out you are on birth control. You get all your Depoprovera shots at Planned Parenthood.

8. **After the first shot, *6 months ago*, you had:**
   - Moderate bleeding (3–4 pads/day) every month.
   - The bleeding would last about 2 weeks.

   After the second shot, *3 months ago*, you had:
   - Light bleeding (2 pads) for 5 days during the first month.
   - No bleeding since then.

- **Pap tests**
  - You got your first Pap test in this clinic when you turned 20 years old at the encouragement of your mother.
  - You had the last Pap done 6 months ago when you started the Depoprovera.
  - Both Pap smears came back normal.

If the student suggests that you can get your shots and your Pap tests done in this office OR asks you why you're going to Planned Parenthood— depending on your level of trust—you can let the student know that you're still on your parents' health insurance and that you don't want them to know about the shots or the tests—or the results of the tests. (See the following for other scenarios around the issue of *trust*.)

SEXUAL HISTORY
Your boyfriend

You've been dating your boyfriend, Chris, who is Caucasian, for the past *8 months*. One of the reasons your father doesn't like Chris is because he is not Latino. The other reason neither of your parents is happy about your dating him is that he's not Catholic. He's a non-practicing Protestant. Your parents made such a fuss over not wanting you to date Chris that you said you would stop seeing him. You have actually continued to see him, but now you're just not telling your parents.

You met Chris in one of your graduate courses. He is also a psychology student who has just started working on his master's degree. He is 22 years old. He lives in an apartment with a roommate. He works at Starbucks.

- Chris is your first sexual partner.
  You don't know how many partners he has had, but you suspect he might have had other girlfriends.
- How often do you have sex? **"Whenever we can."** (That amounts to two or three times a week.)
- Do you ever stay overnight at his place?
     "Are you kidding. I'm expected to be home. That's one of the reasons I want to be able to get my own place."

- You and Chris use condoms "... **most of the time**" (meaning 95% of the time).
- You have NEVER had any sexually transmitted diseases.
- You have NEVER been pregnant.

The way that you handle any of these issues when they come up should indicate to the student that something else is going on. Remember, you don't want your parents to find out that you are still seeing your boyfriend.

Concerns about pregnancy
- If the student asks you if you think you might be pregnant, BEFORE finding out that you are sexually active OR on Depoprovera, you answer straightforwardly, **"No, I don't."**
- If the student asks you if you think you might be pregnant, AFTER finding out that you are sexually active OR on Depoprovera, you waffle, wondering if there's any chance that you might be pregnant, then make up your mind that you're not, finally questioning the student:

    "Noooo ... (hesitate) I don't think ... No, I'm not pregnant ... (pause) **Do *you* think I'm pregnant?"**

When the student suggests that you *might be pregnant* and that s/he needs to do a *pregnancy test,* your response should be in this order:

1. *Worried and anxious* over the possibility of being pregnant. You can reiterate that you are on Depoprovera and that you and Chris use condoms. If the student convinces you that pregnancy is a real possibility, or that the pain means you might have an ectopic pregnancy (a life-threatening condition), your mind becomes flooded with thoughts of what this will mean—even to the point of starting to cry.
2. *Concerned and fearful* that the insurance company will send a statement to your parents indicating that you not only had an office visit, but that you had a pregnancy test.

Here is a diagram of Maria's primary concerns and the decisions you will have to make depending on the student's approach to the topics of sexual activity, birth control, and your last menstrual cycle:

Primary Concerns of Maria Gomez

⇒   Confidentiality of medical record regarding her sexual activity
⇒   Privacy of information/insurance company notification to her parents

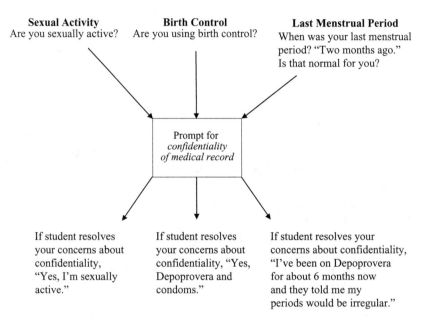

Sexual Activity
Are you sexually active?

Birth Control
Are you using birth control?

Last Menstrual Period
When was your last menstrual period? "Two months ago." Is that normal for you?

Prompt for *confidentiality of medical record*

If student resolves your concerns about confidentiality, "Yes, I'm sexually active."

If student resolves your concerns about confidentiality, "Yes, Depoprovera and condoms."

If student resolves your concerns about confidentiality, "I've been on Depoprovera for about 6 months now and they told me my periods would be irregular."

Maria brings up her concern about the *insurance company notification* to her parents only under the following circumstance(s):
   • If the student orders a pregnancy test
          AND/OR
   • If the student orders a test for sexually transmitted diseases (STDs)

If the student is *not* convincing in how s/he handles the medical record/insurance company issues, you tell the student:

> **"You know, I don't think I'm pregnant and I don't think I need the STD tests, so I don't see any reason why I need to have them done."**

If the student pushes the issue, you can end the conversation by simply saying:

> **"OK, I'll get the tests done at Planned Parenthood."**

THE PATIENT'S LIFESTYLE/HABITS

Alcohol

You drink a glass of wine when you eat dinner out with Chris on the weekends. You never drink in front of your family.

Tobacco

You have never smoked.

Caffeine

You drink a cup of coffee in the morning, then have 4 to 6 diet cokes during the rest of the day.

Diet

You try to eat low fat, fast food meals (salads at McDonald's or chicken sandwiches). You do like french fries and hamburgers and have them at least a couple times a week. You have dinner at home pretty much every night except when you have a night class. The meals at home are prepared by your grandmother and she cooks Mexican food.

Exercise

You don't get much exercise. Occasionally you and Chris go bike riding or take walks together, but you don't consider yourself physically active.

Activities/Hobbies

When you are not studying, you hang out with your friends, go shopping and to the movies. You and your friends also like to find inexpensive, really good ethnic food restaurants.

Stress

If the student asks you whether you have been under any stress lately, you can talk about the stress of living at home and hiding your relationship with your boyfriend as well as the stress of graduate school and working part-time.

FAMILY HISTORY/SOCIAL HISTORY (blood relatives)

You and your family were born in Guadalajara, Mexico. Your immediate family came to [insert city] 16 years ago when you were 5 years old. Your paternal grandparents still live in Mexico. All of you visit Guadalajara at least once a year.

Your father is 47 years old. He is an engineer working for [insert company name]. You have a respectful relationship with both of your parents. He has strong ideas about what he wants for you. You used to fight him when you were a teenager, but now you listen politely and then do what seems right to you when you're not in his presence.

Your mother is 46 years old. She is Director of the Day Care Center at St. Elizabeth's Catholic Church. She's had a struggle balancing raising you and your sister and working as an administrator. She has high hopes for both of you, seeing you married well and having grandchildren for her to dote on as she gets older.

You still talk with your Mom about many things going on in your life, but you don't tell her anything about your sex life OR about anything that might cause her to worry OR that would compromise her situation in the family as "the-good-wife-who-supports-her-husband."

Both of your parents believe education is the best way for their daughters to get ahead. They want to see you finish graduate school before you get involved with anyone. You interpret this as wanting you to put your life "on hold" and follow their ideas about how you should live.

Nothing you tell your parents seems to affect the way they view things. They are still treating you as if you were a teenager. You think this is partly because you are still living at home. The only reason you are living at home is to save enough money to be able to get an apartment of your own so you don't have to feel like you're still a kid. What your parents don't understand is that you do want to finish your graduate degree, but you want to "have a life" at the same time that you are working and going to school. You do not believe, as your parents do, that if you date—or marry—a non-Latino that you will lose your cultural heritage.

Your sister, Lupe, is 17 years old and a senior in high school. She's planning on going to college next year if she gets in. You and Lupe are close, share everything, so Lupe knows what you are keeping secret from your parents.

Your grandmother, Lola, is 72 years old. She stays at home, cooks, gardens, sews, and generally takes care of the home for the rest of your busy family.

Sunday—Family Day: Because yours is such a busy middle class family with everybody leading active lives, Sunday has become the day that the whole family is expected to spend time together. After going to Mass, everyone is expected to have breakfast together and then hang out doing various activities either around the house, or going to a movie, or handling various chores. Whatever the activity is, it must be a "family" activity.

FAMILY MEDICAL HISTORY
Both of your parents and your sister are currently healthy with no medical problems. Your grandmother Lola has diabetes that she controls with diet and exercise.

PERSONAL HISTORY

Living arrangements

You still live at home with your parents, but are planning to move out as soon as you've finished your master's degree.

Education

Right after you got your bachelor's degree you immediately started working on a master's in psychology. You want to be a marriage, family, child counselor (MFCC). You've always had an interest in human behavior and want to help families communicate better with each other. (Maria's motivation stems from her own family situation—and she's aware of that.)

Occupational history

You work part-time as a sales clerk at a clothing store called [insert name of store].

Health insurance

You are covered by your parent's Blue Cross medical insurance. You paid a $20.00 co-pay for today's visit.

Religion

Your parents and grandparents are Roman Catholic. They insisted that you go to a Catholic college. Lupe has decided she wants to go to [insert name of local secular college] and is constantly arguing with her parents over her choice. She's applied to both Catholic and secular colleges just to appease them.

Although you go with your parents to church every Sunday, you are a Catholic in name only. Your parents are not aware of your internal feelings about religion. They just wouldn't understand.

To Roman Catholics, premarital sex is a mortal sin. Pregnancy before marriage brings dishonor to the whole family. Throughout the time you were growing up, your Dad would tell both you and Lupe that he would throw you out of the house if you ever got pregnant before you were married. He's adamant about his views. There's no room for discussion. He knows what's right. He's the father. He sets the rules and expects everyone to follow them.

You told your parents about Chris when you first started dating him, but because your Dad reacted so negatively about your dating someone who is non-Catholic and White, you pretended to listen and have continued to see Chris without your parents knowing it. The only one in your family who knows the truth is your sister.

PHYSICAL EXAMINATION

The student should explain to you what s/he is doing during the physical exam. You are not in excruciating pain; therefore, any necessary shifts in position have little effect on your pain level.

*The student should **begin** the checklist portion of the physical exam of your abdomen by making sure you are lying on your back, then:*

Listening: The student must listen with a stethoscope in *any quadrant BEFORE doing anything else* in order to get credit for doing this correctly on the checklist.

SIMULATION: **You need do nothing except lie still. If the students *press hard* with the stethoscope in the *area of pain* (suprapubic area—just above your pubic bone), you should let them know that you can feel the pain.** There is no need to wince or make faces.

After listening to your abdomen, the student can proceed in any order with the following:

Pressing/Palpating: This maneuver consists of the student touching you with the flat part of their fingers. S/he should start *away from the site of your pain* and press in *all four quadrants* to get credit for doing this checklist item correctly. The student should start pressing your abdomen *lightly* and then press *harder* with their fingertips (this should cause a visible skin indentation).

SIMULATION: **The pain is "crampy" and you just feel it more when the students press on this area, either with the stethoscope or with their hands. All you need to do is *say* that you can feel it more when they *press lightly* in that area (mild tenderness); and that you feel *slightly more pain* when they *press deeply*. But the pain is not enough to ever cause it to show on your face.**

Your belly should remain soft throughout the exam. In other words, do not "guard"(tighten) your lower abdominal muscles.

The student may press on your abdomen and ask if it hurts where s/he is pressing or in any other area. *It hurts when s/he is pressing where you already have the pain.* Nowhere else.

Peritoneal/rebound tenderness: The student might press his/her fingers firmly and slowly into your abdomen (in any quadrant) and then quickly release them. S/he should watch and listen for signs of pain OR ask you whether pressing or letting go hurts more OR to show him/her exactly where it hurts.

SIMULATION: **You will feel the pain more when the student *presses in* on the area of your pain than when s/he lets go. If the student does this rebound maneuver in any other area of your abdomen, there is no difference in the pain.**

In order to check your pain, the student may do either of the following: bump into the exam table OR hit the heel of your foot with his/her fist. Neither of these maneuvers will cause any increase in your abdominal pain.

Rectal/pelvic exam: The student should ask to do a pelvic exam OR a bimanual exam OR a Pap test/smear.

SIMULATION: Tell the student, **"The results of that test are in a folder** [indicate where in the room the student can find them.]**"**

If the student asks if a Pap smear has been done, you respond:
"I'm not sure, but they did do a pelvic and the results are in the drawer." The student should receive credit for this item on the checklist.

DEALING WITH OPEN-ENDED QUESTIONS and GUIDELINES FOR DISCLOSURE

1. You may freely give general information about such "cultural" issues as your parents' expectations for you and your religion as soon as the student starts talking about your family.

   On subjects you don't want your parents to find out about, Only Give Details AFTER the student has dealt with your concerns about **confidentiality** and your **medical record**.

2. Another way a student might try to understand what is going on with you is to encourage you to **say more about your symptoms:** "Can you tell me more about your pain?" OR "What else can you tell me about the symptoms you're having?"

   In this specific circumstance, *you may let the student know* that the *pain has been constant since it started 2 days ago.* (**See Item #2 on the checklist.**)

Checklist

Maria Gomez

OVERALL SATISFACTION (OS)

1. As Maria Gomez, rate your overall level of satisfaction with this student encounter.

   - Outstanding
   - Very Good
   - Good
   - Needs Improvement
   - Marginal
   - Unacceptable

HISTORY (HX)
The student asked me

2. whether the pain is *constant* OR if it comes and goes. ("The pain has been there since it started.")

   - Yes
   - No

3. if the pain *goes anywhere* else. ("No. It's just here in the middle.")

   - Yes
   - No

4. if anything makes the pain *better-or-worse* [Must ask BOTH]. ("Nothing really.")

   - Yes
   - No

5. if I have felt *nauseated* OR *vomited.* ("No, I haven't.")

   - Yes
   - No

6. **about my *bowel habits*.** ("Nothing's changed. I go once a day.")
   o Yes
   o No

7. **about my *bladder habits* OR how often I have to urinate.** ("I have to go a lot more often, like every hour or two.")
   o Yes
   o No

8. **if I have *pain* OR *burning* on urination.** ("Yes—for about 3 days now.")
   o Yes
   o No

9. **to describe my *vaginal discharge* OR color OR amount OR odor.** ("It's white. I'm having a lot more in the past couple days. There's no odor.")
   o Yes
   o No

10. **if I have noticed any *blood* in my urine.** ("No. My urine's yellow.")
    o Yes
    o No

11. **when my *last menstrual period* began.** ("It was about 2 months ago.") [See Training Materials for when to discuss Depoprovera.]
    o Yes
    o No

12. **found out that I am *sexually active*.** ("Does everything I tell you go in my medical record?" If student gives satisfactory answer, then "Yes.")
    o Yes
    o No

13. **if I have 3 (OR more) of the following *HIV risk factors*:**
    – Number of partners I have had: "One."
    – Number of partners my boyfriend has had: "I don't know."
    – Are you in a monogamous relationship? "Yes, I think so."
    – Blood transfusion: "No."
    – IV drugs/STDs: "No."
    – Condom use: "We use them most of the time—like maybe 95%."
    o Yes
    o No

14. what *medications* I am taking. ("None.")

     ○ Yes
     ○ No

15. found out that I am using *birth control*. ("Depoprovera shots and we use condoms.")

     ○ Yes
     ○ No

16. if I have been *physically* OR *emotionally harmed* by anyone. ("No way.")

     ○ Yes
     ○ No

PHYSICAL EXAM (PE)
The student

17. made sure that I was *lying on my back* during the abdominal examination.

     ○ Done
     ○ Not Done

18. *listened* to my abdomen in at least *one* place (*before* touching my abdomen).

     ○ Done
     ○ Not Done
     ○ Done Incorrectly

19. *pressed* on my abdomen. (Must press lightly AND deeply in four quadrants, starting in the upper quadrants away from the pain.)

     ○ Done
     ○ Not Done
     ○ Done Incorrectly

20. asked to perform a *pelvic exam.*

- Done
- Not Done
- Done Incorrectly

INFORMATION SHARING (IS)
The student

21. effectively addressed my concerns about *confidentiality* (around my medical records OR identification of lab tests on insurance company statement).

- Yes
- No

22. counseled me on the *use of condoms* to prevent STDs.

- Yes
- No

CLINICAL COURTESY (CC)
The student

23. *introduced* him/herself to me (must use last name AND title).

- Yes
- No

24. *washed hands* before the PE.

- Yes
- No
- N/A

25. *explained in advance* on at least *one* occasion what s/he would be doing during the physical examination.

- Yes
- No
- N/A

26. *conveyed* at least one aspect of the *results* of the physical examination to you.

  o Yes
  o No
  o N/A

27. respected or looked out for your *comfort.*

  o Yes
  o No
  o N/A

28. *appropriately draped* you during the PE.

  o Yes
  o No
  o N/A

PATIENT/PHYSICIAN INTERACTION (PPI)
(Adapted with permission from East Tennessee State University-Common Ground Rating Form)
**Outstanding should be used only for the few students who do something out of the usual.
*Unacceptable is used only for the few students who leave an unusually bad impression.

The student

29. **appeared professionally competent** – seemed to know what s/he was doing; inspired my confidence; appeared to have my interests at heart.

  o Outstanding
  o Very Good
  o Good
  o Needs Improvement
  o Marginal
  o Unacceptable

30. **effectively gathered information** – collected information in a way that seemed organized; began with several open-ended questions and progressed through interview using a balanced ratio of open- to closed-ended questions; summarized periodically.

  o Outstanding
  o Very Good
  o Good
  o Needs Improvement
  o Marginal
  o Unacceptable

31. **listened actively** – paid attention to both my verbal and nonverbal cues; used facial expressions/body language to express encouragement; avoided interruptions; asked questions to make sure s/he understood what I said.

   o Outstanding
   o Very Good
   o Good
   o Needs Improvement
   o Marginal
   o Unacceptable

32. **established personal rapport** – introduced self warmly; verbally/nonverbally showed interest in me as a person, not just my condition; avoided technical jargon.

   o Outstanding
   o Very Good
   o Good
   o Needs Improvement
   o Marginal
   o Unacceptable

33. **appropriately explored my perspective** – encouraged me to identify everything that I needed to say.

   o Outstanding
   o Very Good
   o Good
   o Needs Improvement
   o Marginal
   o Unacceptable

34. **addressed my feelings** – acknowledged my personal feelings and experience; made statements (verbal or nonverbal) expressing empathy and support.

   o Outstanding
   o Very Good
   o Good
   o Needs improvement
   o Marginal
   o Unacceptable

35. **met my needs** – worked toward a plan that addressed both the diagnosis and my concerns about my illness.

- o Outstanding
- o Very Good
- o Good
- o Needs Improvement
- o Marginal
- o Unacceptable

COMMENTS

Case Summary
From the Patient's Perspective

Maria Gomez thinks she might have a bladder infection because that's what her friend, who had similar pain, was diagnosed with. However, during the course of the interview, she becomes fearful and anxious if the student convinces her that (despite the birth control measures she's taken) she needs to have a pregnancy test—or other tests to rule out sexually transmitted diseases. In addition to what these possibilities could mean for her future, Maria is worried that her parents will find out that she is sexually active. She needs the student doctor to (a) demonstrate competence in figuring out what might be causing her pain; (b) create an atmosphere of trust so she feels comfortable sharing her concerns; (c) validate and show empathy for her worries; and (d) reassure her that her parents cannot see her medical records unless she consents.

Begin your comments with this sentence:

As Maria Gomez, I felt . . .

Guide to the Checklist

Maria Gomez

Item #1:   As Maria Gomez, rate your overall level of satisfaction with this student encounter.

> Your response to this item should be as "Maria Gomez"—NOT as you, the person portraying the patient who knows what the student is being tested on in the checklist. The idea behind this item is to determine your overall satisfaction with the encounter immediately after the student leaves the room. It encompasses whether
> - you feel you would come back to this student doctor for the rest of your care.
> - you feel this student was able or will be able to help you (in your total care).

You will be marking the student using one of six categories from *outstanding* to *unacceptable* using the following criteria to determine which one to choose:
- If the student was so exceptional that you would be inspired to write a letter of congratulation to the student's supervisor, mark "**Outstanding.**"
- If you feel your experience with the student was a positive one, choose "**Very Good**" or "**Good.**"
- If you are slightly dissatisfied with the encounter, are not sure whether the student will be able to help you, or disliked the encounter but not enough to keep you from coming back, choose "**Needs Improvement.**"
- If you feel anything in the encounter with the student negatively affected you significantly enough for you to consider seeing someone else for your care, choose "**Marginal.**"
- Finally, if the experience was bad enough for you to want to report the student to his/her supervisor, mark the student "**Unacceptable.**"

** Remember that the "Outstanding" and "Unacceptable" categories are reserved ONLY for the students who are exceptional on either end of the spectrum. You might only experience this kind of student once or twice in an entire assessment period.

It is all right if your response on this item does not add up to the responses you will make on the history, physical exam, or information-sharing items on the checklist. However, there should be some correlation between your response on this item and on how you answer the Patient–Physician Interaction items. This item is included so that you can make a global assessment based on Maria's overall feeling about the encounter right after the student leaves.

**DEALING WITH COMPOUND QUESTIONS
FROM THE STUDENT**

If the interviewer asks *a compound question with more than two items* (for example, "Have you had a problem eating or drinking, had any nausea or vomiting, or eaten anything that might have been tainted?"), use the following guidelines:

Answer only the LAST question asked. (In the previous question, you would respond regarding having eaten anything that was tainted.)

OR

Answer the MOST COMFORTABLE question asked. (If the patient were a drug abuser and was asked, "Do you drink or use drugs?" you might only give information about your alcohol use.)

OR

If the interviewer asks *only two questions and they are easy to remember* (for example, "Have you had any vaginal itching or burning on urination?"), *answer BOTH COMPONENTS SEPARATELY* even if the answer is the same for both items of the question: "No, I haven't had any burning or itching." Do NOT just answer "No" to a dual compound question.

GIVING CREDIT FOR COMPOUND QUESTIONS

Give credit on the checklist ONLY FOR THE QUESTION(S) YOU ANSWERED. If the student does not go back and ask about the other components of a question, *do NOT give credit for them.* The students MUST ask questions in such a way that they know specifically what it is you are responding to.

HISTORY

The student asked me

Item #2:   whether the pain is *constant* or if it comes and goes.

       YES: The student must ask you if the pain is constant OR if the pain comes and goes OR how long the pain lasts OR *an open-ended question like, "Tell me more about your pain."*

       Your response: "The pain has been there since it started."

Item #3:   if the pain *goes anywhere* else.

       YES: To get credit on this item, the student must try to find out if the pain is solely located in the middle of your lower abdomen or if it *radiates* to any other part of your body.

       Your response: "No. It's just here in the middle."

Item #4:   if anything makes the pain *better-or-worse.*

       YES: To get credit on this item, the student must ask BOTH what you do that makes the pain better **AND** what you do that makes the pain worse.

       Your response: "Nothing really makes a difference."

       NO: If the student asks if the pain itself has gotten better or worse *since it started.*

Item #5:   if I have felt *nauseated* OR *vomited.*

YES: The student MUST ask you if you felt nauseated OR if you have vomited. If s/he asks if there have been any changes in your GI system/your digestion, you may respond by asking what the student means.

Your response: "No, I haven't."

Item #6:   about my *bowel habits.*

YES: The student must ask you if you have had any changes in bowel movements OR if you have had diarrhea/constipation OR to describe your bowel habits.

Your response: "Nothing's changed. I go once a day." [See Training Materials for other details.]

Item #7:   about my *bladder habits* OR *how often* I have to urinate.

YES: The student must ask you about your current bladder habits OR changes in frequency of urination.

Your response: (Thinking) "Yeah, I have to go a lot more often, every hour or 2."

NO: If the student only mentions *urgency* and doesn't bring up frequency.

Item #8:   if I have *pain* OR *burning* on urination.

YES: The student must ask you about any problems with urination (burning, pain, hesitancy, etc.).

Your response: "Yes—for about 3 days now."

Item #9:   to describe the *vaginal discharge* OR *color* OR *amount* OR *odor.*

YES: The student must have already found out that you are having a discharge and go one step further—by either asking you specifics about the discharge OR by asking you to describe the discharge to them—in order to get credit for this item.

Your response: Depending on the question the student asks: (Shyly) "It's white. I'm having a lot more in the past couple of days. There's no odor."

NO: If the student asks you if you've had "spotting" or "bleeding."

Item #10:   if I have noticed any *blood in my urine.*

YES: The student must ask you directly about blood OR what color your urine is OR if the color of your urine is pink/red.

Your response: "No, I haven't seen any blood. . . . My urine's yellow."

Item #11:   **when my *last menstrual period* began.**

YES: The student must ask you when your last menstrual period started OR the date of your last menstrual period. (*Be prepared to give a date 8 weeks ago.*)

Your response: "My last menstrual period was about 2 months ago."

Item #12:   **found out that I am *sexually active*.**

YES: The student may find out that you are sexually active by
- finding out that you have a *sexual* partner (not just a boyfriend).
- asking you directly if you are sexually active.
- asking if, or otherwise finding out that, you are using birth control of any sort.

Your response: "Does everything I tell you go in my medical record?"

     If the student answers so that you feel confident in continuing, you can let the student know that you are sexually active.

Item #13:   **if I have 3 (OR more) of the following *HIV risk factors* (number of partners I have had/boyfriend has had; monogamy; blood transfusion; IV drugs; any STDs; use condoms 100% of time).**

YES: *The student must specifically ask about at least three HIV risk factors.*
- "Do you use IV drugs?" or "Do you use injectable drugs?"
- "Have you ever had sex with an IV drug user?"
- "Have you ever had a blood transfusion?"
- "Ever had sex with a bisexual man?"
- "Ever had any STDs?"
- "Do you use condoms 100% of the time?"

Your response: "No" to everything listed above EXCEPT for the question on condom use which you answer: "Not 100% of the time, but most of the time—like maybe 95%."

- "Are you monogamous?"
- "Is your boyfriend monogamous?"
- "How many sexual partners have you had/has your boyfriend had?"

Your responses: "Yes, I'm monogamous. I don't know how many partners Chris has had, but I know that I'm his only girlfriend now."

NO: *If the student simply asks a semi-open-ended, general question such as "Do you have any HIV risk factors?"*

Your response: "I don't think so . . . ."

*NOTE: Because this item relates to HIV *risk* factors, the following types of questions would NOT allow a student to receive credit for this item:
- "Have you ever been tested for HIV?" ("No.")
- "Have you been exposed to HIV?" ("Not that I know of.")
- "Do you have HIV?" ([worried] "No... I don't think so. Is *that* what you think I have?")

Item #14:   what *medications* I am taking.
    YES: Are you on any medications?
             Are you taking any prescription medications?
    Your response: "None."

Item #15:   found out that I am using *birth control.*
    YES: Are you using birth control?
             Are you on birth control pills?
             The student might ask if you are using "protection." (This can mean protection against pregnancy or sexually transmitted infections.)
    Your response: "I'm getting Depoprovera shots and we use condoms."

Item #16:   if I have been *physically* OR *emotionally harmed* by anyone.
    YES: The point of this item is for the student to determine if physical or emotional abuse is the cause of your abdominal pain.
             "Are you ever afraid of your parents? Of your boyfriend?"
             "Would anything bad happen if your parents found out about your boyfriend?"
    Your response: "No way."
    NO: "Are you under any stress?"
             "What's your stress level like?"

PHYSICAL EXAM

General Guidelines:

DONE INCORRECTLY: Mark any item "Done Incorrectly" if the student
1. does not do the maneuver exactly as described in the following.
2. performs any maneuver THROUGH THE FABRIC OF YOUR GOWN.

    **Any time you mark Done Incorrectly, be sure to indicate, in the comment box below the item, what the student did wrong.

NOT DONE: If the student does not attempt the maneuver at all.

The student

Item #17:   made sure that I was *lying on my back* during the abdominal examination.

It is important that you do not move from your sitting position to your back until the student asks you or helps you to do so. When you lie on your back, it does not hurt more to have your legs straight than to have them bent.

DONE: The student should ask you to lie on your back OR ensure that you are lying on your back before proceeding with the abdominal examination.

NOT DONE: If the student makes no attempt to place you on your back, you should stay sitting. The student gets no credit for this checklist item.

Item #18:   *listened* to my abdomen in at least *one* place *before* touching my abdomen.

DONE: The student must *listen* with a stethoscope in any *quadrant* BEFORE *doing anything else* in order to get credit for this item.

DONE INCORRECTLY: If the student listens *after* s/he has performed any of the other abdominal exam maneuvers.

NOT DONE: If the student makes no attempt to listen to your abdomen at all.

Item #19:   *pressed* on my abdomen (must press *lightly AND deeply* in all 4 quadrants starting in the upper quadrants away from the pain).

DONE: The student should start *away from the site of your pain* in the upper quadrants and palpate/press in **all four quadrants** to get credit for this item. The student should start pressing your abdomen *lightly* and then press *harder* with his/her fingertips (this should cause a visible skin indentation). The student may press all 4 quadrants lightly, then press all 4 quadrants deeply OR start pressing lightly and go deeply as s/he moves from quadrant to quadrant.

Your response:

- You feel slight pain when the student presses lightly in the area where you feel the crampy pain; slightly more pain when the student presses harder.
- Do NOT wince.
- Keep your belly soft throughout the exam.
- If, while pressing on the area right above your pubic bone in the center of your abdomen, the student asks if that makes you feel uncomfortable or as if you have to go to the bathroom, your answer is "Yes." Do NOT volunteer this information, wait for the student to ask.

DONE INCORRECTLY: If the student does not perform the maneuvers as described OR does not press both *lightly and then deeply* in *all four quadrants* OR does not start in the upper quadrants *away* from the site of the pain.

NOT DONE: If the student makes no attempt to press on your abdomen at all.

Item #20: **asked to perform a *pelvic exam.***

DONE: The student must specifically ask to do a pelvic exam OR a bimanual exam OR if one has already been done OR if a Pap smear has been done AND must look at the results of the exam.

Your response: Tell the student, **"The results are in the folder in the drawer."**

DONE INCORRECTLY: If the student does not look at the results or attempts to do the exam without asking you.

NOT DONE: If the student did not ask to do a pelvic exam at all.

INFORMATION SHARING

The student

Item #21: **effectively addressed my concerns about *confidentiality.***

YES: The student needs to directly discuss your desire not to have certain information included in your medical records. The student needs to convince you of his/her point of view (no matter what it is) so that you *feel comfortable* about sharing the concerns you have about *birth control, being sexually active, your fear that you might be pregnant AND that your parents might find out about these private, personal matters.*

> For example, if the student feels the need to record everything in the medical record, s/he needs to *convince* you that your parents will not be able to look at your medical record without your consent OR the student needs to work with you to figure out some way for you to have/get the tests you don't want your parents to find out about (STD and pregnancy tests) from the billing statement sent to them by Blue Cross insurance. The student can do this in any way that makes you feel comfortable to proceed with having the tests.

The point is that the student needs to address your concerns about confidentiality in such a way that you feel assured that your parents will not find out about the pregnancy test or anything else to do with your sexual activities and boyfriend.

Item #22:   counseled me on the *use of condoms* to prevent STDs.

    YES: The student should find out what you know about condom use and then provide more information as needed.

CLINICAL COURTESY

Please record whether the student did the following during the physical exam (PE):

Item #23:   *Introduced* him/herself to me (must use last name AND title).

    YES: If the student tells you his/her last name and his/her title AT ANY TIME during the encounter.

    NO: If the student does not tell you BOTH his/her last name and title.

Item #24:   *Washed hands* BEFORE the PE.

    YES: You must see the student actually wash his/her hands, OR use antibacterial gel, OR s/he must put on gloves before doing the PE.

    N/A: If the student did not wash, use gel, or glove his/her hands because s/he did not do a physical exam at all.

Item #25:   *Explained in advance* on at least *one* occasion what s/he would be doing during the physical examination.

    YES: The student explained at least one time what s/he would be doing EITHER before starting the PE OR before doing one or another of the maneuvers: "I'm going to be doing a heart exam on you" OR "I'm going to check your eyes with a light" OR "I'm going to test the sensation in your legs now."

    NO: If the student is too vague. "Now I'm going to do a physical exam."

            If the student merely asks you to follow directions: "Please hold your head still while you are following my finger with your eyes."

            If the student asks you to describe what you are feeling: "Does it hurt when I press here?" OR "Can you feel this?"

    N/A: If the student did not do a physical exam at all.

Item #26:   **Conveyed at least one aspect of the *results* of the physical exam to you.**

YES: If the student tells you what s/he has found (heard, saw, felt) EITHER *during or after the completion of the PE.* The point here is that the student talks to you about what s/he discovered when doing the physical exam. ("Your lungs sound fine" OR "Even though you're feeling pain right here, I don't feel anything unusual.") The intent is for the student to respect you enough to keep you informed about what s/he is finding as the exam progresses.

NO: If the student does not tell you what s/he has found either during or after the PE.

N/A: If the student did not do a physical exam at all.

Item #27:   **Respected or looked out for your *comfort.***
              *Remember: this item is about your *physical* comfort. (Emotional comfort is covered in the PPI.)

YES: The student did not hurt you during the exam/was not unnecessarily rough OR apologized for hurting you and then adjusted his/her touch OR explained why it was necessary to do a particular maneuver that causes discomfort during the examination OR other behavior such as apologizing for cold hands, offering you Kleenex, and so on.

NO: The student was unnecessarily rough AND offered no explanation OR continued in the same fashion even after you indicated that s/he was hurting you OR ignored other ways during the encounter to make things physically or emotionally easier.

N/A: If the student did not do a physical exam at all.

Item #28:   **Appropriately draped you during the PE.**

YES: If the student covers you with a sheet for the abdominal exam maneuvers and only reveals the area of the body s/he is examining. It's okay to examine your heart and lungs with your gown down.

NO: If the student does not drape you as just described.

N/A: If the student did not do any physical exam at all.

PATIENT/PHYSICIAN INTERACTION
(Adapted with permission from the East Tennessee State University-Common Ground Rating Form)

> Throughout this PPI section, you are to answer each item on the following 6-point Likert scale: **OUTSTANDING, VERY GOOD, GOOD, NEEDS IMPROVEMENT, MARGINAL,** or **UNACCEPTABLE.** You will be indicating your best estimate of how *completely* the student accomplishes the objectives of a given item.
>
> - If the student was so exceptional that you would be inspired to write a letter of congratulation to the student's supervisor, mark "Outstanding."
> - If you feel your experience with the student was a positive one, choose "Very Good" or "Good."
> - If you are slightly dissatisfied with the experience OR are not sure whether the student accomplished the objective of the item OR you disliked what the student did enough to flag his/her behavior, choose "Needs Improvement."
> - If you feel anything in the encounter with the student negatively affected you significantly enough for you to want the student to get remedial help, choose "Marginal."
> - Finally, if the experience was bad enough for you to want to report the student to his/her supervisor, mark the student "Unacceptable."

**Remember that the "Outstanding" and "Unacceptable" categories are reserved ONLY for the students who are exceptional on either end of the spectrum. You might only experience this kind of student once or twice in an entire assessment period.

The student
#29.   appeared professionally competent.
- Seemed to know what s/he was doing.
- Inspired my confidence. (I felt I could trust the student because of the student's own level of self-confidence.)
- Appeared to have my interests at heart.

#30.   effectively gathered information.
- Collected information in a way that seemed organized.
- Began with several open-ended questions (e.g., "What brings you in. . . ?" "Tell me more." "Anything else you are concerned about?") and progressed through the interview using a balanced ratio of open- to closed-ended questions.
- Summarized periodically.

#31. listened actively.
This item has to do with your sensing that the student understands what you are putting out verbally and/or nonverbally (anxiety, fear, embarrassment, why you don't feel you can follow a particular regimen, etc.). It does NOT have to do with effectively dealing with what the student senses is going on with you. *Effectively dealing with this information* should be handled in the ***addressed feelings*** item [Item #34].

- Paid attention to both my verbal and nonverbal cues.
- Used comfortable eye contact, facial expressions, nodding, pauses, posture and body language to express encouragement.
- Avoided interruptions. (It is important to distinguish between supportive interruptions and interruptions that "cut you off.")
- Asked questions to make sure s/he understood what I said.

#32. established personal rapport.
- Showed interest in me as a "person," not just in my condition.
- Introduced self warmly.
- Addressed me by name.
- Used nonverbal expression of interest (warmth in tone of voice, eye contact, body language, etc.)
- Used verbal expression of interest (social interest; personal, supportive or collaborative comments).
- Used understandable language; did not use unexplained technical jargon.

#33. appropriately explored my perspective.
Encouraged me to identify everything that I needed to say.
If the student does not find out how you are experiencing your situation, your expectations, your views on the problem/illness AND how you feel about what s/he is suggesting for the next steps in your care, the student cannot fully meet your needs [Item #35]. (This item [#33] and the "Met my needs" item [#35] work in tandem.)

- Determined my reason(s)—both stated and unstated—for the visit.
- Explored the reason for the patient's clues (if any).
- Explored for unexpressed feelings.
- Inquired about my ideas, my concerns, my expectations about the illness.
- Encouraged me to ask questions.

#34. **addressed my feelings.**
Expressed interest in my personal feelings and experience.

- Acknowledged my personal feelings and experience (which were expressed verbally and/or nonverbally).
- Made me feel understood by using specific statements of empathy and support.
- Validated, legitimized, and/or normalized my medical concerns and feelings.

#35. **met my needs.**
Worked toward a plan that takes into consideration both the student's diagnosis and treatment plan (the student's perspective) as well as your concerns about your illness and follow-up care (your perspective).

- Clearly explained diagnostic and/or therapeutic plan.
- Gave me some sense of
  1. what s/he thought was going on with me.
  2. the anticipated course of the illness.
  3. what was going to happen next.
- Included my concerns in the treatment plan.
- Provided me with choices/options regarding my care.
- Negotiated with me to come to a mutually agreeable plan (e.g., checked to see how I felt about the plan).

COMMENTS

Case Summary
From the Patient's Perspective

Maria Gomez thinks she might have a bladder infection because that's what her friend, who had similar pain, was diagnosed with. However, during the course of the interview, she becomes fearful and anxious if the student convinces her that (despite the birth control measures she's taken) she needs to have a pregnancy test—or other tests to rule out having sexually transmitted diseases. In addition to what these possibilities could mean for her future, Maria is worried that her parents will find out that she is sexually active. She needs the student doctor to (a) demonstrate competence in figuring out what might be causing her pain; (b) create an atmosphere of trust so that she feels comfortable sharing her concerns; (c) validate and show empathy for her worries; and (d) reassure her that her parents cannot see her medical records unless she consents.

Begin your comments with this sentence:
As Maria Gomez, I felt...

Remember that all comments are to be made from the point of view of Maria Gomez—NOT as you, the person portraying the patient who might have a different personality, lifestyle, values and/or attitudes.

As an aid to capturing your feelings, you might want to create a short list of adjectives/descriptors that you can use to complete the opening phrase of the comment section: "As Maria Gomez, I felt . . ."

> When making positive comments, the list you create might include words such as "cared for," "understood," "heard," "confident," "relieved," "satisfied."

> When making constructive comments, your list might include words such as "disregarded," "unimportant," "uncertain," "irritated," "talked down to."

In the document, "Guidelines for Giving Written Feedback," you will find suggestions to help you with writing comments. Included in that document are some general reminders about giving feedback, as well as several Maria Gomez case-specific suggestions (under Key Responses) that you can use if you are having trouble finding ideas or subject matter to write about.

APPENDIX A 6

Guidelines for Giving Written Feedback

Maria Gomez

1. **Jot down trigger words.**
   Take notes as you are filling out the PPI items. These notes will help you remember and sort out what you want to share with the student.

2. **Use information in the "From the Patient's Perspective" case summary.**

3. **Use the "club sandwich" technique.**
   At the beginning, in the middle, and at the end of the feedback, write positive comments about the student's performance.

4. **Let the student know how "Maria" felt.**
   Describe how the student's behavior affected you *as the patient Maria.*

5. **Describe specific student behavior(s)** that caused Maria to respond either positively or negatively toward the student.
   - If the student's behavior *positively affected* Maria, *reinforce the student* by describing specifics of the student's behavior that had a positive effect on her.
   - If the student's behavior *negatively affected* Maria, *suggest another approach* the student might have taken to improve communication with her that will help the student more effectively handle similar situations in the future.

6. **Use these Key Responses:**
   If you are having trouble coming up with ideas, select two or three topics from the list below:

   - Help the student to understand that Maria is *not going to talk* about anything she doesn't want her parents to know *unless the student discusses confidentiality* with her first.
   - Discuss how her shyness makes it *difficult for Maria to talk about sexual matters.* Let the student know what s/he might have done to make it easier for Maria in this regard.
   - Let the student know if there was anything specifically that s/he could have done to *ease Maria's anxiety about the possibility of being pregnant.*
   - Share with the student why Maria is *so afraid* that her parents' *insurance company might notify them* that she had *pregnancy/STD tests* done.

7. **Use the Overall Satisfaction Item.**
   Using checklist item #1, conclude your comments by straightforwardly letting the student know

   - if you would come back to him/her for the rest of your care.
   - if you feel s/he was or will be able to help you.

Pelvic/Rectal Results

Maria Gomez

Here are the findings for the pelvic and rectal exams you just performed on Maria Gomez:

Pelvic Exam:
External genitalia: no redness of the skin or lesions.
Vagina: slight white discharge in the vaginal vault; no fishy odor.
Cervix: no discharge; no cervical motion tenderness.
Uterus: mild fundal tenderness with palpation; no masses felt.
Adnexa: no masses or tenderness.

Rectal Exam:
The anus appears normal on inspection.
On digital examination, there is normal sphincter tone.
Small amount of brown stool in the rectal vault that is heme negative.
No masses found.

Interstation Exercise

Maria Gomez

Write the Assessment and Plan sections of a SOAP note on Maria Gomez.

Assessment

Plan

Interstation Exercise Key

Maria Gomez

Write the Assessment and Plan sections of a SOAP note on Maria Gomez.

Assessment

1. 21 y/o G0P0 with lower abdominal pain—relatively benign exam. Consider UTI, PID, R/O pregnancy. Doubt appendicitis.
2. Family stressors.

Plan

The student should order the following laboratory tests:

1. Urinalysis (dip and spun for microscopic evaluation)
2. Wet mount for bacterial vaginal discharge
3. KOH for yeast infection
4. Urine pregnancy test
5. Cervical cultures for gonorrhea and chlamydia
6. HIV test

Audition Case Summary

Maria Gomez

Maria Gomez is a 21-year-old Latina who has come to the doctor's office because of stomach pains that she has been experiencing for the past 2 days. She is a college student starting to work on her master's degree. She lives at home and is still covered by her parents' health insurance. She does not want her parents to know that she is sexually active or, if it comes up in the clinical encounter, that she might be pregnant, or even to know that she is still dating the boyfriend they disapprove of because he is neither Latino nor Catholic.

Presentation/Emotional Tone

Maria is a pleasant young woman; however, she is shy and guarded when talking about her sex life. She will answer the doctor's questions, but is embarrassed if asked to elaborate with details. In other words, the doctor has to "help" her talk about her sexual activities. She is most comfortable if the student doctor just asks her questions to which she can simply give one-word answers.

Changes in Demeanor During the Encounter

At the beginning of the encounter, as the patient you think you might have a bladder infection because that's what your friend, who had similar pain, was diagnosed with. However, during the course of the interview, you become afraid and anxious if the student doctor convinces you that (despite the birth control measures you've taken) you need to have a pregnancy test—or other tests to rule out sexually transmitted diseases. You can reiterate that you are on birth control and that you and your boyfriend Chris use condoms. If the student convinces you that this is a real possibility, or that the pain means you might have an ectopic pregnancy (a life-threatening condition), you become flooded with thoughts of what this will mean—even to the point of starting to cry.

The student should sense you want to talk about something that is disturbing you. If s/he responds to your emotion by letting you know everything that goes on between the two of you is *confidential*, you respond:

"(Hesitating) **Look, my parents didn't want me to be dating my boyfriend, so when they objected I pretended that I broke up with him, but I'm still seeing Chris. Both my parents, but my Dad in particular, only want me to date Latino Catholic boys and** *not* **until after I finish my education. Chris doesn't fit their idea of who I should be seeing.**"

History of Present Illness

When you woke up a couple of days ago, the pain was mild. It has not gone away since you first noticed it. In fact, it has gotten slightly worse.

Reason for Clinic Visit

> When the student asks what brings you in to the clinic today, you respond:
> "**I've had this crampy pain in the middle of my stomach for the last 2 days. I noticed it right here** (gesture with the flat palm of your hand in the middle lower abdominal area when you say this) **when I woke up a couple of days ago.**"

Pain Symptoms

- **Better or worse** – Nothing makes the pain better or worse. In other words, it's not any better if you're sitting, standing, or lying down.
- **Intensity** – On a scale of 1 to 10, with "1" being a barely noticeable pain and "10" being the worst pain you've ever experienced, *this abdominal pain started out a "2" two days ago and has increased to about a "4" now.*
- **Other pain questions**
  Any other questions about the pain (that are not on the accompanying checklist you got with this summary), you answer in the negative. For example, the pain:
  – Does NOT wake you up at night.
  – Does NOT interfere with your normal activities.

Other Symptoms

The student may ask you if you've experienced any of the following:

- **Changes in eating habits** – None.
  You have been able to eat normally for the past 2 days. You had nothing unusual to eat the night before you woke up with the pain.
- **Increase in urinary frequency** – You notice that you *are* having to "go to the bathroom" more frequently.
- **Vaginal discharge** – You are embarrassed to talk about this. If the student simply asks if you are having a vaginal discharge, you only say: "**Yes, I am . . . .** until they ask other questions.

- **Vaginal bleeding** – Not in the past 2 days. Only when you're having your period.
- **Pain with intercourse** – (If the student hasn't found out that you have a boyfriend and are sexually active, hesitate, look a little embarrassed and concerned, then nod and say: "**I** *am* **having some pain . . . .**" The pain with intercourse has been only in the past 2 days.)

Menstrual History

You are not comfortable talking about this subject or about birth control; therefore, you only answer whatever the student asks. For example, When was your last menstrual period? "**Two months ago.**" Are your periods irregular? "**They have been lately.**" How long have they been irregular? "**Since about 6 months ago.**" Did anything happen 6 months ago that caused them to become irregular? "**I started getting birth control shots.**"

Family History

You and your family were born in Guadalajara, Mexico. Your immediate family came to [insert city] when you were 5 years old. All of you visit Guadalajara at least once a year to see your relatives.

Your father has strong ideas about what he wants for you. You used to fight him when you were a teenager, but now you listen politely and then do what seems right to you when you're not in his presence.

Your mother has had a struggle balancing raising you and your sister, Lupe, and working. You still talk with your Mom about many things going on in your life, but you don't tell her anything about your sex life OR about anything that might cause her to worry.

Your sister, Lupe, is 17 years old and a senior in high school. She's planning to go to college next year if she gets in. You and Lupe are close, share everything, so Lupe knows what you are keeping secret from your parents.

Audition Abridged Checklist

Maria Gomez

HISTORY (HX)

The student asked me

1. whether the pain is *constant* OR if it comes and goes. ("The pain has been there since it started.")

   o Yes
   o No

2. if the pain *goes anywhere* else. ("No. It's just here in the middle.")

   o Yes
   o No

3. if I have felt *nauseated* OR *vomited.* ("No, I haven't.")

   o Yes
   o No

4. about my *bowel habits.* ("Nothing's changed. I go once a day.")

   o Yes
   o No

5. about my *bladder habits* OR how often I have to urinate. ("I have to go a lot more often, like every hour or 2.")

   o Yes
   o No

6. if I have *pain* OR *burning* on urination.("Yes – for about 3 days now.")

   o Yes
   o No

7. to describe my *vaginal discharge* OR color OR amount OR odor. ("It's white. I'm having a lot more in the past couple days. There's no odor.")

   ○ Yes
   ○ No

8. if I have noticed any *blood* in my urine. ("No, my urine's yellow.")

   ○ Yes
   ○ No

9. found out that I am *sexually active.* ("Does everything I tell you go in my medical record?" If student gives satisfactory answer, then "Yes.")

   ○ Yes
   ○ No

10. found out that I am using *birth control.* ("Depoprovera shots and we use condoms.")

    ○ Yes
    ○ No

PHYSICAL EXAM (PE)
The student:

11. made sure that I was *lying on my back* during the abdominal examination.

    ○ Done
    ○ Not Done

12. *listened* to my abdomen in at least *one* place (*before* touching my abdomen).

    ○ Done
    ○ Not Done
    ○ Done Incorrectly

13. *pressed* on my abdomen. (must press lightly AND deeply in four quadrants, starting in the upper quadrants away from the pain.)

   o Done
   o Not Done
   o Done Incorrectly

14. asked to perform a *pelvic exam.*

   o Done
   o Not Done
   o Done Incorrectly

INFORMATION SHARING (IS)
The student

15. effectively addressed my concerns about *confidentiality.*

   o Yes
   o No

16. counseled me on the *use of condoms* to prevent STDs.

   o Yes
   o No

APPENDIX B

Standardized Patient Administrative Forms

Sample
Letter of Agreement

Date
SP's Name
Address
City, State, Zip Code

Dear [SP name]:

Thank you for agreeing to participate as a Standardized Patient in the Clinical Practice Exam (CPX) to be administered at the [name of institution]. We are pleased to inform you that you have been selected to perform the [case name] patient case.

Let me quickly reiterate in writing what we have discussed informally with you in terms of dates of participation and payment for your work. Much of the success of this exam depends on your full participation and commitment. Please carefully review the following:

TRAINING

Your training will consist of a series of four training sessions and a Practice Exam, for which you will be paid a total of $___ . You will do Sessions One, Two, and Three with your trainer. Session Four will be a "dress rehearsal" with you performing your patient case with a faculty physician. Session Five will be a Practice Exam similar to the actual exam administrations in which you will participate. All of the SPs portraying your patient case will be present with you at all four of the training sessions and the Practice Exam.

The focus of your first training session will be familiarization with the detailed training materials and checklist for your case. A summary of what will take place during the rest of training will be discussed at this first session, which will last about 3 hours. The other training sessions will last between 3 and $3\frac{1}{2}$ hours each.

All of the practice encounters in the training sessions will be video recorded for possible review by the CPX advisory committee. It is this committee that will determine if your performance in the portrayal of the case and the accuracy of your checklists meets CPX committee standards. If, at any time during your training or performances, the committee determines that your work is not meeting these standards, you may be terminated.

All standardized patient cases at [name of institution] are the property of the [name of institution]. By participating in the [name of institution] program, and by accepting payment for training and performance of any [name of institution] cases, you are agreeing not to perform these cases anywhere else unless specifically requested to do so by [name], Director, [name of SP Program], [name of institution].

LOCATION FOR TRAINING

All training sessions will be held at: [name of institution, address, building, and room number].

Parking permits will be provided.

EXAMINATION/PERFORMANCE

You must be available every day between [list month, inclusive dates, and year]. You must be present at the [name of building and location within building] for the morning administration from [inclusive times] or for the afternoon administration from [inclusive times]. The exact days and times for your performances will be scheduled with your coach during the third training session. During the days when you are not performing, please plan to be "on call" until 7 p.m. the evening before.

PAYMENT

You will be paid $___.00 for each exam administration in which you participate. Your invoice will be submitted to [name of institution] on the last day of your performance. You can expect payment for both training and performances approximately 6 weeks from that date.

CONSENT

Carefully review this letter. If you agree to all the terms, please sign both copies. Return one to your coach at your first training session. Keep the other copy for your files. If you have any questions, please feel free to contact [coach's name or assistant] at [telephone number].

My colleagues and I look forward to seeing you again and working with you on this interesting and challenging project.

Sincerely,

[Standardized Patient Program director's name, director's title]

SP AGREEMENT:

I hereby agree to the above terms and performance schedule. I also agree to participate in the four training sessions and the Practice Exam to be held during the months of _____ and _____. In addition, I confirm that I do not have a relationship with, nor do I have contact with, any medical student at [name of institution].

Signature: _____

[Type in SP's name]

Standardized Patient Profile Form

1. Name (as it appears on Social Security Card):_____
2. Home Address:_____
   _____
3. Phone and E-mail Information:
           Home: ( )_____ Mobile:_____
           Work: ( )_____ E-mail:_____
4. Date of Birth:_____
5. Height:_____
6. Weight:_____
7. Ethnicity:_____
8. Country of Birth:_____
9. Languages Spoken:_____
10. Education (circle one)   High School   College: Year 1 2 3 4
        Highest Degree Completed_____ Area of Study_____
11. Have you ever had surgery?_____
12. Do you have scars or other physical findings that may be detected during a physical examination (such as surgical scars, skin piercings, tattoos, heart murmurs, or chronic conditions, for example asthma, arthritis, high blood pressure, diabetes, etc.)?

   _____
   _____
   _____

(For Office Use Only)

Auditioned for:
    Case(s)   Program   Date

_____
_____

Comments:

Sample
Recorded Image
Consent-and-Release Form

I hereby give my permission, without reservation or restriction of any kind, stated or implied, to [name of institution], to photograph me in still, digital, film, or video formats, or any combination thereof.

I further consent and authorize that all such produced and derived material in which I appear may be used by [name of institution] in any manner whatsoever for all and/or any purposes for medical use, instruction, demonstration, or exhibition, public or private.

Further, I consent, without reservation or restriction of any kind, stated or implied, that all such produced and/or derived material may be distributed and/or circulated by [name of institution] wherever to whomever they may deem necessary or desirable for any general or specific educational uses.

Further, I hereby waive any right to compensation for these uses, and I release from all or any liability, now and forever [name of institution], its directors, officers, employees, agents, and students from and against any claim for injury or compensation resulting from the activities authorized by this agreement.

Signature of SP:_____ Date:_____

Print Name:_____

Witness:_____

Index

Believability (*continued*)
Blindness, simulation of, 23
Body, sensations and internal feeling states,
    55–57, 96–97, 102–103
Breathing control
    in emotional state portrayal, 56, 57
    in pain portrayal, 96–97
    and performance anxiety, 92
Brook, Peter, 60, 61, 87

C

Cancer, portrayal of, 121,
    190
Candidate notification, 146–147
Candidate recruitment. *See*
    Recruitment
Carnovsky, Morris, 7, 8
Carotid bruits, simulation of, 23
Case familiarity, coping with, 201
Case materials
    analysis of, 53–54, 62–67
    Gomez case study, 269–325
    pre-audition, 125, 134–137, 139
    in training, 160, 166–168
    writing, 5
Case portrayal. *See also* Patient portrayal
    familiarization (*See* Training Session
        One)
    inside-out approach, preparation for,
        62–75
    overview, 40–41, 246
    performance of, 78–81 (*See also*
        Performances)
    standardization in, 46
Casting
    auditions (*See* Auditions)
    experienced SPs, 117, 118
    overview, 9–11, 40, 109
    recruitment (*See* Recruitment)
    resources, 135–136
Challenge, Standardization of case, 46,
    104–105
Cheat sheets, 194–195, 205–206
Checklists. *See also* Information disclosure
    guidelines
    accuracy goals, achieving, 3–4, 184–186,
        191–193, 198–202, 212–213,
        247–248, 252–254, 259–261
    activities, 167–168, 187–193
    for auditions, 137, 139, 141–143
    for coaches, 237–238

coaching principles, 17, 19–21,
    184–186, 210–212, 245, 246
Gomez case study, 291–297, 323–325
and information disclosure, 34, 171
keys for videos, 175, 191
overview, 25, 27, 28, 183–184
physical examination, 172–174
protocol for, 35–37, 204
recollection and, 35
satisfaction item, 222–223
saving, 188–189
Clarification, requesting in information
    sharing, 34
Clinical practice examination (CPX)
    administrative details, 208–209
    advisory committee (*See* CPX advisory
        committee)
    guidelines, 256
    overview, 4–5, 218–219
    preparation for, 196, 239, 246–247,
        256–258
    standardization in, 46–47
    training session overview, 161
    validation of authenticity for (*See*
        Validation of authenticity)
Clinical skill areas, knowledge acquisition
    in, 17, 36–38
Clinical skills assessment. *See also* Clinical
    practice examination (CPX)
    open-ended questions, 30
    SPs in, 5, 6, 11–13, 141
Clinicians
    in authenticity checking, 25, 156,
        173
    recruitment of, 175–176
    in SP training, specialists, 176
    in training sessions, 203–204, 228,
        230–236
"Club Sandwich" Technique, 221
Coaches. *See also* Directing the SPs
        performance
    and acting/directing, 43–50, 83
    as actors, 206–207
    overview, 7–9, 259–262
    preparation
        CPX, 257–258
        Practice Exam, 241
        training sessions, 175–176, 194–196,
            214–215
    qualities of, 7–9
    skills required, 3–5, 13–14, 37–38

Medical issues, not discussing, 220. *See also* Information disclosure guidelines

Medical students
  as actors, 10
  assessment of, 5–7, 9, 23–24, 26, 112–114, 183–184
  communication skills required by, 27–29, 215–216
  education of, 3, 4, 17–19, 25
  and experienced SPs, 117
  feedback, receiving, 216–219
  information sharing/education skills, 32–34
  listening by, 78–79
  observation of, 12–13, 114
  patient response to, 77, 200
  portrayal of, 31, 34–36, 42, 46, 171, 206–207

Medicare documentation requirements, 26

Memory
  affective, 73–74
  in character portrayal, 52, 72
  and concentration, 79, 186
  of facts, 180–181
  and feelings, 58, 101–103
  recollection skills, 35, 114, 185, 186, 193, 201–202
  in recruits, 114

Mental disorders, portrayal of, 51, 120

The Method described, 42. *See also* Stanislavsky, Constantin

Monitoring, 240–241, 252–254. *See also* Observation skills

Motivation, 42–43, 52, 53, 68–72, 180

Moulage in simulation, 23, 214

Muscle weakness, simulation of, 23

N

Needs of the patient in acting performances, 42

Newspapers/newsletters in recruitment, 119–120

Note-taking, 210–211

O

Objectives in acting performances, 68–72

Objectivity, 217

Observation skills
  in clinicians, 232
  medical students, 12–13, 114
  PPI, 27, 233, 245
  Practice Exam, 250–252
  protocol during Practice Exam, 228, 250–252
  protocol during Training Session Four, 228
  in recruits, 12–13, 114
  in SPs, 236–237, 246

Olivier, Lawrence, 52

On call requests, 164. *See also* Availability

Orientation of examinees, 254

Outline of the Training Procedures (OTP), 158, 159, 160

Outside agencies, recruiting through, 118–119

Outside-in approach to believability, 50–60

P

Pain, portrayal of, 94–97

Parking issues, 164

Parkinson's Disease, simulation of, 23

Patient education skills, 32–34

Patient perspective
  on the checklist, 186
  coaching, 168–169, 216
  discovery of, 30–31, 40
  and feedback, 219–220, 223–224
  Gomez case study, 297

Patient–physician interaction (PPI)
  as a resource for SP comments, 223
  on the checklist, 186, 218–219
  and information sharing, 32–33
  observation of, 27, 233, 245
  overview, 26–32

Patient–Physician Interaction (PPI) scale, 28

Patient portrayal. *See also* Authenticity; Case portrayal; Standardization
  case materials analysis and, 62–67
  enhancement of, 50–51, 216
  guidelines, 47
  imagination in, 72–75
  living as the patient, 179–180
  motivations/intentions/objectives in, 68–72
  overview, 11–12, 211, 212
  patient's psyche, getting into, 39–41

SPRINGER PUBLISHING COMPANY

Intuition and Metacognition in Medical Education

Keys to Developing Expertise

Mark Quirk, EdD

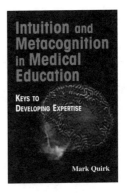

From Mark Quirk, a 2006 Society of Teachers of Family Medicine's Excellence in Education award recipient, comes the latest on improving medical education.

In this volume, Quirk explores the idea of metacognition, the idea that we can think about the way we or other people think and thus gain a better understanding of ourselves, our own cognitive processes, and the patients we seek to help. Written for medical educators—from medical school faculty to the most self-reflective residents—this book will help you teach your students and interns how to extrapolate lessons from experience and integrate learning and practice. It will help them to think more clearly and thoroughly about what they read, hear, and learn on a day-to-day basis and thus become more informed and humanistic doctors.

Partial Contents:

An Emerging Paradigm for Medical Education • Developing Expertise as the Aim of Medical Education • Metcognitive Capabilities • The Role of Intuition • Clinical Expertise: A Blend of Intuition and Metacognition • Clinical Problem Solving • Communication and the Physician-Patient Relationship • Professionalism • Teaching Expertise • Self-Directed Learning • A New Curricular Paradigm for Medical Education

2006   174pp   0-8261-0213-1   hardcover

11 West 42nd Street, New York, NY 10036-8002 • Fax: 212-941-7842
Order Toll-Free: 877-687-7476 • Order On-line: www.springerpub.com